Your Last Diet

A Journey to Wellness

Austin Spruill, M.D., Ph.D.

License to reproduce "The Diet Readiness Questionnaire" was obtained from The National Academies Press and Copyright Clearance Center.

Permission to use the worksheets for "Relapse Prevention" was kindly granted by the Kaiser Permanente Center for Health Research.

Grateful acknowledgement is made to Dr. Eric Westman for allowing me to use his "No Sugar, No Starch" Diet plan with my patients.

Published by Austin Spruill
Cover Design by Nathaniel Dasco
Edited by Asher Spruill

If we treat people as they are, we make them worse. If we treat people as they ought to be, we help them become what they are capable of becoming.

— Johann Wolfgang von Goethe

Table of Contents

Introduction

Not Another Diet Book

I know what you are thinking: *NOT ANOTHER DIET BOOK!* Don't worry—this is *not* just another diet book. Hopefully, this will be the *last* "diet" book you ever buy! This book was written to get people off the diet treadmill and onto a path of health and wellness beyond just losing weight. If you just want a plan to lose weight there is a plethora of books out there that can tell you how to lose weight. However, this book challenges the "diet mentality" and focuses instead on getting healthy and staying healthy. Making the necessary changes to become and stay healthy can be intimidating and seem overwhelming. Whether you need to lose weight or make adjustments in your lifestyle in order to live longer, this book helps navigate that process in a stepwise fashion. My recommendations are designed to guide you from *losing weight* to *healthier eating and living*. If you read this book and apply these recommendations, then you will find yourself walking the path of lasting success in your personal wellness journey.

Many people need help on this journey; they need a guide, a roadmap to reverse the course they are on. Their lives may even depend on making a course correction. Perhaps that's you, but all you can think of are the obstacles in your path.

Do you lack access to weight loss programs, fitness centers, or gyms?

You will discover as you read on that it is possible to lose weight and get healthier on your own. It can be done. Many people have done it. You just need to be armed with information, given some tools, and have someone join you on your journey to keep you on track. Sometimes the hardest part of the journey is planning and packing. This book will not only help you with the planning and packing, but also provide a roadmap for your journey. Once you have a clear vision for the journey, you can start on the path toward your destination—living a healthier, longer life.

Have you tried a number of diets or weight-loss programs and had success, only to gain the weight back?

There are so many diets and approaches that yield weight loss. However, the challenge is maintaining weight loss. Undoubtedly, this is the greatest challenge in obesity medicine today. It is generally true that over 90% of people who lose weight gain it back. Weight loss, however, is not the end goal; long-lasting health is. Sustained lifestyle changes are essential to sustained weight loss and wellness. This program will not only help you lose weight but teach you how to maintain your weight loss.

Do you hate to exercise? Do physical limitations hinder you from exercising?

You've been told, *eat less and exercise more*, and you are miserable, right? Guess what—you can lose weight and improve your health without exercising. This wellness program enables you to eat more and exercise less and lose weight. I am not saying that exercise is not important, but I am saying that it is not required to achieve significant weight loss and improve health. During the initial phase of the wellness program the activity recommendations are intended to jump start rapid weight loss. The latter part of the book promotes regular exercise during the transition from dieting to a healthier lifestyle in order to achieve sustainable changes.

Do you need to lower your blood pressure, reverse type 2 diabetes, or improve your cholesterol numbers? Does your weight bring you physical, emotional, or spiritual pain?

Join the many women and men who have overcome weight-related health problems by following the recommendations in this book. If you apply these recommendations you should see your health improve and experience reversal of some of the disorders associated with being overweight. Wouldn't you like to get off some of the medications you are taking?

Have you or someone you know been diagnosed with cognitive impairment or dementia?

Consuming a low-inflammatory diet, as well as taking certain nutraceuticals can help to improve cognitive function. Whether you need to lose weight or not, this book provides low-inflammatory nutritional plans and recommendations for maintaining brain health.

Are you thinking, I don't have any weight-related issues, but I would like to learn how to eat healthier and live longer?

If that's you, keep reading because there are sections in the book that will help you make lifestyle changes to improve your overall health and enhance your longevity. People everywhere are trying different diets to achieve different health benefits. The key for everyone seeking lasting health—whether they struggle with their weight or not—is to make lifestyle adjustments, and not just dietary changes. Part Two of this book focuses on embracing a healthy lifestyle.

A True Story

Let me tell you a real life story about a couple who had some weight-related problems and decided to break free from the "diet mentality." J.M. enrolled in my program at age 53 and was accompanied by her husband at her first visit. They both had lost some weight on their own prior to this visit. However, she needed to lose more weight to be able to get a hip replacement. She was in constant pain and unable to exercise. Her husband had been recently diagnosed with type 2 diabetes mellitus and was on medication for high blood pressure. They decided that he would adopt the same diet as his wife. After two weeks in the program, his blood sugars had normalized, and by six weeks he had discontinued his blood pressure medicine. At that point J.M. had begun to start doing some light aerobic activity. After about 15 weeks she had lost almost 40 lbs., and he had lost almost 50 lbs. Her hip surgery the following month brought complete recovery of function. They visited me four months later, and she had lost an additional 40 lbs. They had joined a gym and were exercising regularly. She had lost a total of 80 lbs. since starting the program, and her BMI had dropped from 38.6 to 24 in about eight months! In addition, her husband had maintained his weight loss.

What was the key to their success? At their initial interview I asked her, "Why are you here today?" She went on to describe the diet treadmill she had been on for most of her life, and said she was ready to be done with it. She had a conviction that her life needed to change. She and her husband wanted lasting change. They were ready to embrace both a new mindset and a new lifestyle.

How about you? Are you ready to break free of the "diet mentality" and adopt a healthy "lifestyle mentality"?

Part I

---

*Breaking Free of the
Diet Mentality*

Chapter One

Preparing for Your Journey

Getting on the path to sustainable weight loss and wellness requires an all-in mindset, a roadmap (this book!), and a traveling companion—someone to support you and keep you on track. I have designed a program to enable you to partner with others who can join you on your journey and provide some accountability so you will not only lose weight but also improve your health and live longer.

It is never too late to make a change. It all starts with the conviction that change is necessary. Perhaps you're sick and tired of the "diet treadmill." Or maybe it's the physical pain or the emotional pain caused by the weight you carry. Maybe it's being faced with life-shortening health conditions.

What will it take for you to "burn your boat" and go all-in with a life-altering wellness program?

"Burn the Boats"

History records accounts of famous military leaders, including Hernán Cortés and Alexander the Great, who, after landing in the countries they intended to invade, ordered their men to *"Burn the boats."* What was the strategy behind this command? They wanted to eliminate any possibility of retreat, and therefore secure unwavering commitment to their mission. It created a "no turning back" attitude. That same mentality is required if you truly want to achieve sustainable lifestyle changes. You don't have to be defined by your past. Instead, break free from your past and embrace a future of health and wellness. You too can adopt a no retreat-type of commitment for yourself.

The couple I shared about in the Introduction "burned the boats" at the beginning of their journey. They bagged up all their large size clothes and donated them to the Salvation Army. No retreat; no regret. Since then they haven't looked back.

Once you make the decision to forget the past and move forward, I am here to help. Perhaps you are wondering, "What am I committing to?" Keep reading. I have a plan for you.

Seven-Step Program to Change

First, I want to give an overview of the *why* of the wellness plan. I'll then outline the *how*. If you don't know why you are doing something it is very difficult to stick with it. There will be times in this journey when you will ask yourself, *"Why am I doing this?"* The more you understand the *why* upfront, the better your chances are for success.

Trust me — you will have to revisit the *why* periodically. The journey will be long and demanding, but if you stay focused on your purpose, your destination — your *why* — you will find the stamina you need.

Step One: Mentality Shift

This wellness program is not a weight-loss or exercise program, but rather commitment to changing your lifestyle—a lifestyle of wellness. It's about improving your health and wellbeing; for some of you, your life depends on it. People on the diet treadmill are operating with a "diet mentality." They try one diet or weight-loss program after another, hoping each one will be the last. Been there, done that? This is such a frustrating cycle. It is emotionally and financially draining. Breaking free from this endless cycle requires a paradigm shift from a "diet mentality" to a healthier "lifestyle mentality." It is not easy, but it is worth it because the payoff is improved health and longevity. The people who make this necessary shift are the ones who succeed. Guaranteed! The most successful patients I have treated, who not only lost weight but also achieved sustained improvement in health, all embraced a "lifestyle mentality." They left the "diet mentality" behind and reaped the long-term benefits.

Step Two: Personal Responsibility

The most enduring lifestyle changes occur when people fully commit to a life-altering decision. These are people like J.M. and her husband from the Introduction. Irv Brechner, the author of *The Mind Diet,* calls it arriving at the Moment of Truth.[1] These are people who resolve to change and then move forward without looking back. Patience, persistence, and perseverance are essential to successfully transform and sustain a lifestyle. Take for example people who have successfully quit smoking. Often when I ask ex-smokers how they did it, they say they just decided to quit and went "cold turkey." It was painful at first, but then it got easier. They simply decided to commit to change. It has to be the same with losing weight and getting healthy. Otherwise, success will be temporary at best. It is about taking personal responsibility for your health. This program is designed to empower you to do exactly that.

Step Three: Healthy Nutrition

The nutritional approach in this program involves eating whole foods and avoiding meal substitutes (such as shakes and bars). There are a number of these weight-loss products on the market, but it can be challenging to transition off meal substitutes during the weight maintenance phase. Alternatively, learning how to purchase and prepare nutrient-rich whole foods will ease the transition and enhance the likelihood of achieving sustainable lifestyle changes. The nutritional plan for weight loss is designed to control hunger and provide a protein-enriched, reduced-carbohydrate, high fat diet that will reverse the metabolic processes that lead to excessive weight gain and associated disorders. Changes in nutrition and eating patterns are necessary for you not only to lose weight, but, more importantly, to sustain weight loss.

Step Four: Exercise

For too long people have been told that the answer to their weight problem is to *"eat less and exercise more."* While this approach may provide some temporary benefits, it often does not produce sustainable weight change. Calorie restriction diets generally leave people hungry and prove very challenging for most people. On this program people can lose weight without exercising. I have had patients with physical limitations due to orthopedic problems who couldn't exercise initially. While performing only minimal activity, they were able to lose extraordinary amounts of weight. As they lost weight and their orthopedic conditions improved, they began to incorporate more activity or exercise into their wellness program.

Regular, consistent activity is essential to sustainable lifestyle changes. The activity recommendations in this book will vary depending on whether a person is in the weight-loss phase or weight-maintenance phase and will take into consideration any physical limitations. Everyone is encouraged to introduce activities to their daily lifestyle to reduce sedentary activity. The recommended activities are designed to increase non-exercise activity thermogenesis (NEAT), which has been shown to assist in weight loss.[2] In brief, you can increase the number of calories your body burns on a daily basis with only a moderate increase in general physical movement.

Step Five: Accountability

Let's face it; left to our own devices we tend to drift back to our old habits. It is human nature. We want to please self. It is hard to say "No" to self, because self is so demanding! It is helpful to have someone come alongside and ask you how you are doing, give you a "high five" when you are successful, or "speak the truth in love" and help you get back on track when you stumble. Perhaps this is a parent, spouse, friend, teacher, pastor, or coach. We all need others to travel beside us and encourage us, especially in a wellness journey like this. The most successful participants in the quest for wellness have traveling companions. Plus, frequent follow up is essential and enables the wellness physician to tweak the program to fit the need of each patient. There is something about having to come in to an office and climb on the scale and be measured that pushes people to try their hardest. Alternatively, it may be checking in online to report self-measurements that provide the needed accountability. Even after reaching the maintenance phase it is important to have ongoing follow up, though less frequently, in order to provide needed accountability.

Step Six: Controlling Personal Environments

Environment is *so* important. Long-term success depends on a prescriptive plan that teaches you to control your personal environment. You need strategies that anticipate challenging situations. So what are the important environments that need attention, and what are some strategies you should consider?

1. **Home**

    -   Start with the point of contact: the grocery store. Shop the perimeter of the store.[3] The foods you need to be eating are found mostly on the perimeter.

    -   Get savvy at reading Nutrition Facts labels. Note the carbohydrate/sugar content.

    -   Stop buying "low fat" items. Fats are not the problem.

    -   Limit technology usage in the home to help avoid sedentary activities known to be associated with increased caloric intake.

2. **Work**

    -   Reduce sedentary activity and increase your NEAT. This keeps your metabolism revved up during the day.

- Get up and move around intermittently, take the stairs, go for a walk during lunch, and park further away from work (as long as it is safe).

- Consider using a standing desk at work or a treadmill desk if you work from home.

- Prepare diet friendly lunches and snacks. The weekends are a great time to plan and prepare your meals for the week.

- Establish a plan to avoid consuming unhealthy foods or beverages available at work (e.g. vending machines, break room).

- Be preemptive by having a strategy when you know there are going to be special celebrations or luncheons.

3. **School**

   - Prepare healthy foods and beverages to take to school because healthy (i.e. diet-friendly) lunches or snacks are generally not an option. Prepare these in advance to enable you to have variety in your diet.

   - Opt out of school lunches. This will reduce the temptation to go off diet when confronted with other dietary choices.

   - Commit to not obtaining unhealthy foods or beverages while at school. Stay away from vending machines.

4. **Dining Out**

   - Preview menus online for diet-friendly options.

   - Order diet-friendly foods and exercise portion control.

- Take leftovers home.

- In the beginning, avoid buffet restaurants.

- Avoid fast food restaurants if possible.

- Ask the waiter not to put bread or chips on the table.

- Substitute salads for forbidden sides. Be careful of dressing content.

- Order water instead of a sweetened beverage.

5. **Vacations**

- Pack diet-friendly foods and beverages.

- Cook as much as possible and limit eating out.

- When eating out go to places with diet-friendly options.

6. **Holidays and Celebrations**

- If you are well into your nutrition plan and having success, then taking a holiday will probably not derail you. You have to know yourself in this regard.

- If you do take a holiday, moderation is the operative word. Moderation means the indulgence can only be a holi*day*, not a holi*week*!

Step Seven: Emotional and Spiritual Support

Humans were created as three-part beings: body, soul, and spirit. In addressing a person's physical state of health, it is important to assess the emotional and spiritual issues that can impact their health. My approach addresses all aspects of a person's life to promote wholeness. Numerous studies have shown the impact of emotional struggles on a person's physical health.[4,5] The effects of stress and negative emotional states on one's weight are well documented.[6] Prayer for physical, emotional or spiritual healing in certain circumstances can be very helpful to facilitate healing or wellness.[7,8] In other cases, assistance may be necessary through counseling to address adverse life events from the past or current crises, since relapse is often associated with these events. The consequences of adverse childhood experiences as they relate to obesity in adulthood are well documented.[9] Lapses are inevitable for most people. Life happens, and when it does there is higher risk for relapse. The goal is to help people weather their lapses so they don't relapse.

The Next Step

Now you have an overview of the wellness plan. The next step is to determine your readiness to undertake this wellness adventure. While readiness is not necessarily a predictor of success, it is a necessary part of preparation for the journey. The next chapter will address readiness.

Chapter Two

Are You Ready?

Before beginning a wellness program, it is important for you to determine your readiness to undertake such a program at this point in your life. I ask all my patients to complete "The Diet Readiness Test" that was originally published by Brownell and utilized by many weight-loss programs.[1] Not only will this test assess your readiness, but it will also help identify potential areas of concern as you proceed with the program.

A copy of the test is found below and was obtained from an Appendix from the Institute of Medicine.[2] There is a scoring guide at the end of each section to assist you in your assessment.

The Diet Readiness Test

Answer the questions below to see how well your attitudes equip you for a weight-loss program. For each question, circle the answer that best describes your attitude. As you complete each of the six sections, add up the numbers of your answers and compare them with the scoring guide at the end of each section.

Section 1: Goals and Attitudes

1. Compared to previous attempts, how motivated to lose weight are you this time?

   1. Not at all motivated
   2. Slightly motivated
   3. Somewhat motivated
   4. Quite motivated
   5. Extremely motivated

2. How certain are you that you will stay committed to a weight loss program for the time it will take you to reach your goal?

   1. Not at all certain
   2. Slightly certain
   3. Somewhat certain
   4. Quite certain
   5. Extremely certain

3. Consider all outside factors at this time in your life (the stress you're feeling at work, your family obligations, etc.). To what extent can you tolerate the effort required to stick to a diet?

   1. Cannot tolerate
   2. Can tolerate somewhat
   3. Uncertain

4. Can tolerate well
5. Can tolerate easily

4. Think honestly about how much weight you hope to lose and how quickly you hope to lose it. Anticipating a weight loss of 1 to 2 pounds per week, how realistic is your expectation?

   1. Very unrealistic
   2. Somewhat unrealistic
   3. Moderately unrealistic
   4. Somewhat realistic
   5. Very realistic

5. While dieting, do you fantasize about eating a lot of your favorite foods?

   1. Always
   2. Frequently
   3. Occasionally

6. While dieting, do you feel deprived, angry and/or upset?

   1. Always
   2. Frequently
   3. Occasionally
   4. Rarely
   5. Never

Section 1 -- TOTAL Score ____

If you scored:

6-16:   This may not be a good time for you to start a weight loss program. Inadequate motivation and commitment together with unrealistic goals could block your progress. Think about those things that contribute to this, and consider changing them before undertaking a diet program.

17-23:   You may be close to being ready to begin a program but should think about ways to boost your preparedness before you begin.

24-30:   The path is clear with respect to goals and attitudes.

Section 2: Hunger and Eating Cues

7. When food comes up in conversation or in something you read, do you want to eat even if you are not hungry?

   1. Never
   2. Rarely
   3. Occasionally
   4. Frequently
   5. Always

8. How often do you eat because of physical hunger?

   1. Always
   2. Frequently
   3. Occasionally

    4. Rarely

    5. Never

9. Do you have trouble controlling your eating when your favorite foods are around the house?

    1. Never

    2. Rarely

    3. Occasionally

    4. Frequently

    5. Always

Section 2 — TOTAL Score ____

If you scored:

3-6:   You might occasionally eat more than you would like, but it does not appear to be a result of high responsiveness to environmental cues. Controlling attitudes that make you eat may be especially helpful.

7-9:   You may have a moderate tendency to eat just because food is available. Dieting may be easier for you if you try to resist external cues and eat only when you are physically hungry.

10-15:   Some or most of your eating may be in response to thinking about food or exposing yourself to temptations to eat. Think of ways to minimize your exposure to temptations, so that you eat only in response to physical hunger.

Section 3: Control over Eating

If the following situations occurred while you were on a diet, would you be likely to eat more or less immediately afterward and for the rest of the day?

10. Although you planned on skipping lunch, a friend talks you into going out for a midday meal.

   1. Would eat much less
   2. Would eat somewhat less
   3. Would make no difference
   4. Would eat somewhat more
   5. Would eat much more

11. You "break" your diet by eating a "forbidden" food.

   1. Would eat much less
   2. Would eat somewhat less
   3. Would make no difference
   4. Would eat somewhat more
   5. Would eat much more

12. You have been following your diet faithfully and decide to test yourself by eating something you consider a treat.

   1. Would eat much less
   2. Would eat somewhat less
   3. Would make no difference
   4. Would eat somewhat more
   5. Would eat much more

Section 3 — TOTAL Score ___

If you scored:

3-7: You recover rapidly from mistakes. However, if you frequently alternate between eating out of control and dieting very strictly, you may have a serious eating problem and should get professional help.

8-11: You do not seem to let unplanned eating disrupt your program. This is a flexible, balanced approach.

12-15: You may be prone to overeat after an event breaks your control or throws you off the track. Your reaction to these problem-causing eating events can be improved.

Section 4: Binge Eating and Purging

13. Aside from holiday feasts, have you ever eaten a large amount of food rapidly and felt afterward that this eating incident was excessive and out of control?

    1. Yes
    2. No

14. If you answered yes to #13 above, how often have you engaged in this behavior during the last year?

    1. Less than once a month
    2. About once a month
    3. A few times a month
    4. About once a week

5. About three times a week
6. Daily

15. Have you ever purged (used laxatives, diuretics, or induced vomiting) to control your weight?

   1. Yes
   2. No

16. If you answered yes to #15 above, how often have you engaged in this behavior during the last year?

   1. Less than once a month
   2. About once a month
   3. A few times a month
   4. About once a week
   5. About three times a week
   6. Daily

Section 4 — TOTAL Score ___

If you scored:

0-1:   It appears that binge eating and purging is not a problem for you.

2-11:   Pay attention to these eating patterns. Should they arise more frequently, get professional help.

12-19:   You show signs of having a potentially serious eating problem. See a counselor experienced in evaluating eating disorders right away.

Section 5: Emotional Eating

17. Do you eat more than you would like to when you have negative feelings such as anxiety, depression, anger, or loneliness?

    1. Never
    2. Rarely
    3. Occasionally
    4. Frequently
    5. Always

18. Do you have trouble controlling your eating when you have positive feelings — do you celebrate feeling good by eating?

    1. Never
    2. Rarely
    3. Occasionally
    4. Frequently
    5. Always

19. When you have unpleasant interactions with others in your life, or after a difficult day at work, do you eat more than you'd like?

    1. Never
    2. Rarely
    3. Occasionally
    4. Frequently
    5. Always

Section 5 — TOTAL Score ___

If you scored:

3–8:   You do not appear to let your emotions affect your eating.

9–11:   You sometimes eat in response to emotional highs and lows. Monitor this behavior to learn when and why it occurs and be prepared to find alternate activities.

12–15:   Emotional ups and downs can stimulate your eating. Try to deal with the feelings that trigger the eating and find other ways to express them.

Section 6: Exercise Patterns and Attitudes

20. How often do you exercise?

    1. Never
    2. Rarely
    3. Occasionally
    4. Somewhat
    5. Frequently

21. How confident are you that you can exercise regularly?

    1. Not at all confident
    2. Slightly confident
    3. Somewhat confident
    4. Highly confident
    5. Completely confident

22. When you think about exercise, do you develop a positive or negative picture in your mind?

    1. Completely negative
    2. Somewhat negative
    3. Neutral
    4. Somewhat positive
    5. Completely positive

23. How certain are you that you can work regular exercise into your daily schedule?

    1. Not at all certain
    2. Slightly certain
    3. Somewhat certain
    4. Quite certain
    5. Extremely certain

Section 6 – TOTAL Score ___

If you scored:

4–10: You're probably not exercising as regularly as you should. Determine whether your attitudes about exercise are blocking your way, then change what you must and put on those walking shoes.

11-16: You need to feel more positive about exercise so you can do it more often. Think of ways to be more active that are fun and fit your lifestyle.

Self-Evaluation

After scoring yourself in each section of this questionnaire, you should be able to better judge your strengths and weaknesses as you begin this journey. A helpful first step in changing eating patterns is to understand the attitudes and conditions that influence your eating habits.

If the scores on your readiness test appear to be favorable at this time in your life, then the next step in your preparation is to see the nutritional plan that is recommended for your wellness journey. The plan that is outlined in the next chapter has been used by countless people to successfully lose weight and reverse weight-related disorders.

Chapter Three

Nutritional Plan for Weight Loss

The nutrition guidelines provided in this plan are adapted from a low-inflammatory, low-carbohydrate, high-fat (LCHF) diet plan promoted by Dr. Eric Westman of the Duke Lifestyle Medicine Clinic, at the Duke University Medical Center. A full description of the diet can be found in his book *The New Atkins for a New You.*[1]

The recommendations in this nutritional plan enable you to change the type of "fuel" you are consuming so that your body will function in a way that will reverse certain metabolic disorders and provide your body with the energy it needs to work efficiently. Erroneous medical information in the 1960s led to the widespread belief that fatty foods caused heart disease.[2] Certain carbohydrates (i.e. sugar and starches) were then promoted as "heart safe." Both the medical profession and the food industry promoted these erroneous ideas, but the subsequent rise in worldwide obesity rates has now caused the medical profession to reevaluate the causes of weight gain. It turns out that the major culprit in this epidemic is the rise in consumption of processed foods and sugar since the 1960s. Our bodies were not designed to handle the amount of processed sugars that many people consume. To correct and reverse weight-related, inflammatory disorders (e.g. type 2 diabetes),[3] the recommended nutritional plan in this chapter reduces carbohydrate intake and increases protein and fat intake.

To achieve effective weight loss and reverse the consequences of unhealthy eating patterns, **your intake of carbohydrates must be limited to 20 grams per day.** This limit will create the necessary "fat burning" effect in the body to reverse the effects of excessive weight gain. During this initial phase of the plan, you will avoid sugar, bread, pasta, fruit, flour, and any other sugary or starchy food or beverage. The nutritional plan gives guidelines for which foods and drinks you can consume and which ones you should avoid during this phase. Following the recommendations in the nutritional plan will help you adjust your eating patterns.

This nutritional plan provides adequate nutrients to meet the metabolic needs of your body and eliminate nutritionally-empty carbohydrates. Only consume the foods and beverages outlined in the following plan. Once you reach your target weight, you will switch to a more sustainable nutritional plan.

Nutritional Plan: Low Carb, High Fat

As mentioned previously, the original source of the diet is Dr. Eric Westman's Lifestyle Medicine Clinic at Duke University Medical Center. The plan described below is an edited version of the "No Sugar, No Starch" Diet published in *Why We Get Fat* by Gary Taubes.[4]

Foods to Eat Daily:

Salad greens: 2 cups a day of arugula, bok choy, cabbage, chives, greens (e.g. turnip, beet, collards, mustard, radish), parsley, endive, kale, lettuce, spinach, or scallions. If it is a leafy vegetable, you may eat it.

Vegetables: 1 cup (uncooked) a day of vegetables like asparagus, broccoli, Brussels sprouts, cauliflower, leeks, celery, cucumber, eggplant, string beans, peppers, mushrooms, okra, onions, shallots, sprouts, snow peas, sugar snap peas, summer squash, tomatoes, and zucchini.

Foods to Eat Often:

Meat: Beef, pork, ham, veal, bacon, lamb, or other meats. For processed meats, check the nutritional label for carbohydrate content which should be about 1 gram per serving. Organic, grass-fed and nitrate-free meats are preferred.

Poultry: Chicken, turkey, or other fowl.

Fish and shellfish: Any fish, as well as shrimp, scallops, lobster and crab are acceptable. Wild seafood is preferred.

Eggs: Whole eggs are permitted.

Foods to Eat in Limited Quantities:

Cheese: You may eat up to 4 ounces a day of aged cheeses such as Swiss and Cheddar, as well as cream cheese, Camembert, Brie, Gruyere, mozzarella, and goat cheeses. The carbohydrate count should be less than 1 gram per serving. No Velveeta.

Cream: You can enjoy no more than 4 tablespoons a day of heavy, light, or sour cream. No Half-and-Half.

Mayonnaise: You may have up to 4 tablespoons a day. Check the labels for carbohydrate content. Duke's and Hellmann's are acceptable.

Olives (black or green): You may have up to 6 a day.

Avocado: You may have half of a fruit a day.

Pickles, dill or sugar-free: You can enjoy up to 2 servings a day. Check the labels for carbohydrates and serving size.

Lemon juice or lime juice: You can enjoy up to 4 teaspoons a day.

Soy sauces: You may have up to 4 tablespoons a day. Check the labels for carbohydrate content. Kikkoman is acceptable.

Snacks: Ham, beef, turkey, pork rinds, pepperoni slices, and deviled eggs are all acceptable snacks.

Daily Menu Template

The following template will help you plan your daily menu:

Breakfast

- Protein source: Meat and/or eggs.

- Fat source: Meat and eggs have fat in them. You can add some fat in the form of cheese, butter, or cream (in coffee). Consider adding a low-carbohydrate vegetable in an omelet or a breakfast quiche to create some variety in your diet.

Lunch

- Protein source: Meat and or cheese.

- Fat source: Meat. Add some fat in the form of salad dressing, avocado, butter cheese, or cream.

- Vegetables: 1 to 1 1/2 cups of salad greens or cooked greens and/or 1/2 to 1 cup of approved vegetables.

Snack

- Protein-enriched, low-carbohydrate snack that contains protein and/or fat to reduce hunger.

Dinner

- Protein source: Meat.

- Fat source: Meat. Add some fat through cream, butter, salad dressing, avocado, or cheese.

- Vegetables: 1 to 1 1/2 cups of salad greens or cooked greens and/or 1/2 to 1 cup of vegetables.

With this nutritional plan, a typical day might look like this:

Breakfast: Bacon and eggs.

Lunch: Salad containing grilled chicken, mixed greens, other vegetables, bacon, chopped eggs, and salad dressing.

Snack: String cheese and/or pepperoni slices.

Dinner: Steak, pork chop, or hamburger with green salad, and other vegetables, such as broccoli or cauliflower with butter.

The daily goal: Protein intake: 12-18 ounces, depending on gender and activity level. Carbohydrate intake: fewer than 20 grams.

Frequently Asked Questions

Why do you recommend this diet instead of another LCHF diet (e.g. South Beach, Zone, Paleo)?

The nutritional plan recommended in this program is based on the Atkins diet that Dr. Atkins first published in 1972 and updated in 2002.[5,6] Drs. Westman, Phinney, and Volek published their iteration of the Atkin's diet in 2010.[1] This diet has been researched extensively and is safe and effective if the recommendations are followed. It has a longer track record and more research supporting its use than any of the other available reduced-carbohydrate diets. Other diets can be effective and may suit a person's particular needs. It has been said that the best diet is the one you can stick with. No matter how effective a diet is, if it doesn't suit the person, it won't work. Many people have found this LCHF nutritional plan suitable for them to achieve their weight loss goals.

Which carbohydrates can I eat on this nutritional plan?

During this phase of the nutritional plan, consume no sugars and no starches.

Sugars are simple carbohydrates and must be avoided. Sugars include: white sugar, molasses, brown sugar, milk, honey, fruit, corn syrup, maple syrup, beer, flavored yogurts, or fruit juice.

Starches are complex carbohydrates and must be avoided. Starches include: grains, rice, cereals, flour, pastas, breads, muffins, bagels, crackers, cornstarch, and "starchy" vegetables such as peas, carrots, corn, potatoes (French fries and potato chips), pinto beans, lima beans or black beans.

The only carbohydrates you should eat during this phase are the nutritionally dense, fiber-rich vegetables listed in the nutritional plan.

Which fats can I eat?

Olive oil and peanut oil are especially healthy oils and are preferred when cooking. Margarine and other hydrogenated oils that contain trans fats should be avoided.

The ideal dressing to use is a homemade oil-and-vinegar dressing. Spices and lemon juice can be added to enhance the flavor. Caesar, ranch, blue cheese, and Italian are also acceptable if their carbohydrate content is only 1-to-2 grams or less. Avoid "low-fat" dressings because they contain too many grams of carbohydrate. Other sources of fats include eggs, bacon, and/or cheese which may be added to salads.

Fats are important to include because they are tasty and filling which reduces hunger. The fat or skin on the meat can be eaten as long as there is no breading on the meat.

Which beverages can I drink?

The best beverage is water. Spring and mineral waters, or essence-flavored (carbonated) waters are acceptable. Occasional beverages with stevia-based natural sweeteners can be consumed.

Caffeine intake can interfere with weight loss and control of blood sugar. Consume no more than 3 cups daily of coffee (black or with approved sweetener and/or heavy cream), and tea (unsweetened or naturally sweetened).

Avoid alcohol consumption on this nutritional plan. Alcoholic beverages often contain sugars; plus, your body burns calories from alcohol first, which delays the fat-burning process. At a later point in time, as your weight loss and dietary patterns become well established, you may add back alcohol in limited quantities. This will be discussed further in later sections of the book.

Do I have to exercise portion control with this plan?

This nutritional plan has an appetite-reducing effect due to the increase in protein and fat intake. Bottom line: Eat when you are hungry. If you are hungry you are probably not eating enough protein. As you will learn, the amount of protein needed will vary from person to person depending on their activity level. This nutritional plan is not about counting calories. If you follow the recommendations in this plan you should lose weight without significant hunger or cravings.

Is timing of meals important for weight loss?

Yes. It is recommended that you start your day with a nutritious protein-enriched meal. The earlier you eat breakfast, the more you accelerate fat-burning and aid your weight loss.[7] Also, the morning protein load will reduce ghrelin, a hunger hormone, and help curb your appetite. Try to establish a schedule of eating three meals a day at about the same time, which will assist greatly with maintaining the plan. A schedule also helps when taking medications and supplements to assist with the weight loss because some medications and nutritional supplements need to be taken before a meal or after having a meal.

How do you read a Nutrition Facts label?

Determine the serving size, and content of total carbohydrate, sugar, and fiber. Focus on the *sugar* content, which is derived by subtracting *dietary fiber* content from *total carbohydrate*. This will enable you to determine your *net carbohydrate count*, which should be no more than 20 grams per day. For example, if the label says there are 6 grams of carbohydrate and 2 grams of fiber, the net carbohydrate count is 4 grams. The net carbohydrate count of vegetables should be less than 5 grams, and 1 gram or less for meats or condiments.

Check the ingredient list and avoid foods that have any form of sugar or starch listed in the first five ingredients, including sucrose, dextrose, maltose, fructose, honey lactose, glucose, agave syrup, molasses, corn syrup, high-fructose corn syrup, maple syrup, corn sweeteners, cane juice, and fruit-juice concentrate.

What else is helpful to know when starting on this plan?

Avoid "diet products" that have "fat-free" or "lite" on their labels. Avoid foods containing hidden sugars and starches (e.g. cakes, sugar-free cookies, and coleslaw). Check the labels of over-the-counter medications that may contain sugar (e.g. antihistamines, cough syrups, cough drops, etc.). Avoid products that are labeled "Approved for Low-Carb Diets!" because many of these products contain too many grams of carbohydrate. Check labels!

Is this nutritional plan a ketogenic diet?

Yes, the body goes into a state of *ketosis* during this initial phase of the nutritional plan because carbohydrate intake is reduced. Ketosis means your body is burning fats in the form of ketones. Ketones result from the breakdown of fat and are a great source of energy. Fat burning is desirable in order to lose weight. Studies have shown ketogenic diets to have multiple health benefits, including increased sensitivity to insulin, lowering of blood glucose levels, positive effects on lipid levels and reducing inflammation.[1] Ketosis also produces neuroprotective benefits which will be discussed in greater detail in a later chapter.[8] You can measure ketones in a urine sample to check to see whether your body has entered a state of ketosis. These strips for testing urine are available over the counter and are easy to use.

Can this nutritional plan be used in children?

Yes, with certain adjustments. Ketogenic diets were first reported in 1920s to be an effective treatment of intractable seizures in children.[9] Some children were kept on these diets safely for several years. One of the reported side effects was weight loss. I have taken care of several children who were put on ketogenic diets because their seizures were not well controlled with anticonvulsants, and they did quite well. I use this nutritional plan as recommended in children older than 12 years old. For younger children, I adjust the carbohydrate limit as needed. The youngest child that I have treated was 5 years old. She weighed 126 lbs. and was already insulin-resistant (insulin level of 57). Her nutritional plan limited her net carbohydrate intake to 50-60 grams each day.

Can vegetarians and vegans use this nutritional plan?

Yes, with certain adjustments. It is recommended[1] that vegetarians consume 30 grams per day of net carbohydrates, and, when increasing carbs back into a vegetarian diet, introduce nuts before berries. It is recommended that vegans consume 50 grams per day of net carbohydrates.[1] This requires including nuts, seeds, and legumes in the diet from the start in order to get sufficient protein. There are very helpful meal plans for vegetarians in *The New Atkins for a New You.*

If I am on medications, do I need to inform my physician that I'm on this nutritional plan?

Medical supervision by your primary care physician (PCP) is recommended during any weight loss program, but especially if you are taking medications. As patients lose weight and their medical conditions improve or resolve, medications will often need to be adjusted or discontinued by their PCP. In particular, if a patient is taking insulin for treatment of type 2 diabetes, and they start on a LCHF diet, their blood sugar levels will drop rapidly. For example, I had a patient who was taking 70 units of insulin a day when they started on the LCHF nutritional plan. At their 1 week follow up they had reduced their dose to 10 units a day, by 2 weeks had reduced their dose to 5 units a day, and by their 1 month follow up they were off insulin. *It is important that you not make adjustments in your medications unless directed to do so by your PCP.*

How important is it for me to drink water while on this plan?

It is very important to drink sufficient amounts of fluid each day (at least 64 ounces) during this phase of the nutrition plan.

Water is preferred, but some non-caffeinated, diet-friendly beverages are permitted.

What do I do if I develop problems with constipation?

Diets with reduced carbohydrate content can lead to constipation. Cell Press, a recommended supplement to take while on the diet, may help with this problem. You may also try Miralax, ColonClenz, or Milk of Magnesia. Doses of these agents will vary, so adjust the amount you take until you achieve the desired effect. The goal is to have one soft stool each day. If the problem persists despite these interventions, discuss this with your physician.

If I experience bad breath while on this diet, what can I do about it?

Some people notice they may have bad breath during the initial phases of this nutritional plan. Drinking plenty of fluids and maintaining good oral hygiene can help this problem. Use Spry gums or mints if needed.

What if I develop headaches, body aches, or feel sluggish when I start this nutritional plan?

Some people starting a reduced-carbohydrate diet can experience transient headaches, body aches, and fatigue. These symptoms are a result of the body changing from burning carbohydrates as fuel to burning fats as fuel. If you experience these symptoms, add one cube of beef or chicken bouillon to a cup of hot water and drink a cup up to three times a day. *Caution: If you have heart failure or high blood pressure, do <u>not</u> consume bouillon.*

What can I do if I crave something sweet?

As you change your eating patterns, it is not unusual to experience cravings for foods that are to be avoided. This is normal; the cravings will pass! Eat a protein snack or a dill pickle, and the craving should diminish.

Can I have low-calorie sweeteners in my diet?

Studies have shown that use of artificial sweeteners is associated with weight gain and increased abdominal obesity.[10,11] This may occur through disruptions in the signaling of the reward system in the brain or through alterations in the composition of the gut microbiome.[11] A recent study reported an increased risk of stroke and dementia associated with consumption of artificially sweetened beverages.[12] Because of these adverse consequences, it is recommended that you avoid using sweeteners. Drink water flavored with lime or lemon juice, but if that is not satisfying, you may use limited amounts of a natural, stevia-based sweetener such as Truvia or Pruvia. Studies are inconsistent on the effects of natural sweeteners on glucose and insulin responses after their consumption. Avoid food or beverages with sugar alcohols (e.g. sorbitol and mannitol) for now. They may be permitted in limited quantities in later stages of your journey.

Should I take vitamins or supplements while on this plan?

Yes. The following supplements are recommended:

- Although limiting carbohydrate intake has been shown to be healthy for children and adults, it is recommended that you take a **multivitamin** (e.g. Centrum or generic equivalent) daily to ensure you are getting all the vitamins and minerals your body needs.

- **Calcium Pyruvate** is recommended to enhance the fat-burning process by accelerating the process of metabolism. **Dose:** 750 mg, 1-2 tablets twice daily (morning and afternoons).

- **Cell Press** is recommended because it has multiple benefits. Cell Press has been found to (i) induce satiety (the sensation of fullness), (ii) reduce constipation, (iii) reduce cravings, and (iv) reduce insulin levels, which helps prevent many of the metabolic consequences of obesity. **Dose:** 1-2 capsules 1 hour before lunch, before supper, and in the evening if hunger becomes an issue between supper time and bed time.

- **Probiotics** have been reported to reduce inflammation and oxidative stress caused by obesity.[13] Because certain strains of *Lactobacillus* and *Bifidobacterium* appear to promote weight loss, reduce gut permeability, decrease inflammatory markers, and decrease metabolic disease markers, their use should be considered in treating weight-related disorders. In particular, the following strains might be beneficial: *L. rhamnosus, L. plantarum, L. gasseri,* and perhaps *L. acidophilus, L. casei, L. lactis, B. bifidum,* and *B. lactis*. **Dose:** 10-20 billion CFU/day for optimal benefits. There are products that contain most or all these strains in a single dose. Check ingredient list if you want to make sure.

These supplements are available online from MyDietShopz.com and Amazon.com.

Before You Begin the Journey

You now have a nutritional plan as your road map and are armed with helpful information; what's next? Before you undertake your wellness journey, careful planning and packing are necessary to ensure success in your endeavor. The next chapter will help with final preparations for your journey.

Chapter Four

Starting Your Journey

You can carry out the wellness program on your own, but to achieve optimal success it is recommended that you involve your physician or enroll in the program online. Let's look at your options.

Option One: Do It Yourself

If you undertake this journey on your own, I would encourage you to do so under a physician's supervision. If you are able, contact the office of your primary care physician (PCP) and arrange to have a physical exam (PE) if you have not had one within the last year. Also, consider having the following labs done before starting the program: Complete Blood Count (CBC), Comprehensive Metabolic Panel (CMP), Lipid Panel, Hemoglobin A1C, Insulin, and Thyroid studies (TSH, T3, and Free T4), C-reactive Protein (CRP), and Vitamin D levels. A baseline EKG is important to obtain if you have known cardiovascular risk factors. Discuss with your PCP whether you need an EKG.

Why is this all necessary? It is helpful to have baseline metrics to monitor the success of the interventions on certain metabolic disorders. PCP involvement is very important if adjustments in medications are required because of weight loss. With this diet blood sugars can drop rather quickly, and insulin dosages will then need to be reduced or discontinued. Blood pressure often normalizes with weight loss, requiring medication dosage reduction or discontinuance.

Option Two: Online Enrollment

Another option is to enroll in the program online to receive personal consultation and accountability from a wellness physician. Intake forms that provide information regarding your medical, family, emotional, spiritual, nutritional, and exercise history need to be completed prior to online enrollment. This information is essential to tailoring the program to your specific needs. The forms are available to download from my website: **roanokewellnesscenter.com.** Also, as part of the enrollment process, patients need to submit a copy of a recent physical exam along with labs performed by their PCP, if they are available. Please contact my office via the website if you are interested in enrolling for virtual consultations.

What to Pack

Supply yourself with all the tools to succeed:

1. A vision

In the Bible, Proverbs 29:18 says, "When there is no vision, the people cast off restraint." When there is no restraint we do whatever seems right for us to do in the moment. A vision, however, enables the question, "Will this action assist me or hinder me in my pursuit of wellness?" Battles are won or lost in the momentary choices. Having a clear vision for wellness provides a lens through which you can assess your choices and keep the big picture in view.

2. A fighting spirit

While a direction-changing decision can be a defining moment in one's life, it is just that: a moment. A single moment doesn't automatically lead to long-term change. However, a series of right choices repeated over time can create sustainable change. Psychologists have studied how long it takes to develop a habit. While it was originally thought it could be done in 21 days, it turns out that it takes on average about two months or more. Therefore, fight those battles of the moment and do what you need to do to stay on track. In time, what you *need* to do will become what you *want* to do. Soon you will be rewarded with sustainable change.

3. Accountability to self

Implement a plan to monitor your progress daily. There are a number of apps for tracking your nutrition, activity, and sleep. (For a list, see the Resources section in the back of this book.) People who track their progress experience greater success. Self-monitoring promotes self-governing, which helps create desired habits. Patience, persistence, and perseverance are essential for personal transformation and maintaining a lifestyle of wellness.

4. Partnership with others

People find it easier to exercise if they have an exercise partner. I have seen this same approach work well for people who want to lose weight. Success is more likely if you are following a wellness program with a family member or friend. Find a wellness "buddy," or even better, form a "wellness group" (e.g. from work, church, school, etc.) to join you in achieving your goal. Create incentives and reward success within your group to make it more fun and to encourage one another in reaching wellness goals. You benefit, and so does everyone else!

5. A "damage control" strategy

Lapses occur as a natural part of weight management. They will happen. However, it is important to identify lapses and intervene before they evolve into a total relapse. There will be bumps in the road, but they don't have to derail you! To prevent lapses, identify situations that are considered high-risk and have a plan to deal with those situations preemptively. This approach is addressed in more detail in the next chapter.

Now that you understand what is required for this wellness plan, what do you need to do to get started?

Final Preparation

Use the following checklist to ensure that you are fully prepared to begin your journey.

- Are your Diet Readiness Test scores favorable to start a wellness program at this time?

- Are you ready to "burn your boat" and commit to a lifestyle change?

- Have you identified someone to support or partner with you in your journey? Or enlisted others to form a "wellness group" to provide mutual accountability?

- Have you had a physical exam and labs performed by your PCP to establish a baseline assessment before starting the program?

- Have you removed all of the forbidden foods and beverages from your house?

- Have you purchased the required diet-friendly foods, snacks, and beverages?

- Have you purchased the recommended supplements and multivitamin?

- Have you arranged for periodic follow up with your PCP or, alternately, enrolled for your follow up online?

- Do you have a set of scales, tape measure, sphygmomanometer (to measure blood pressure), glucometer (to measure blood sugar) if you are going to enroll online?

If you have completed all the above tasks, then you are ready to undertake this life-altering journey. Take a breath and go for it!

Launch Day

Start by obtaining all your baseline measurements: weight, height, chest, waist, hips, thigh; establish baselines for blood pressure, heart rate, respiratory rate and blood sugar (if diabetic). Eat the prescribed foods along with taking your supplements and multivitamin as instructed. Most people lose a significant amount of weight the first week due to fluid shifts as the body adjusts to the dietary changes. The goal is to lose 2-3 pounds per week. This can usually be achieved by adherence to the nutritional plan.

Arrange a follow up visit with your PCP or check in online after one or two weeks to assess your progress. Ideally, you should have weekly or bimonthly follow up visits for two to four months, and then the frequency can be adjusted if you are doing well with the program. **Patients who commit to regular follow up experience greater success.** The accountability provided by frequent visits is crucial during the early phase of the program. It is desirable to reach your target weight as soon possible and then maintain a lifestyle of wellness. The schedule can be adjusted depending on the timeline of reaching health goals.

Reasonable benchmarks for weight loss are 5% by two months, 10% by four months, 12% by six months, and 15% by twelve months. Some people will not reach the benchmarks and others will exceed them. Significant improvement in health of patients with type 2 diabetes occurs when a person loses more than 10% of their weight.[1] This is easily achievable by following the recommendations offered in this wellness program. Two-thirds of my adult patients have achieved greater than 10% weight loss if they continued the program more than 16 weeks.

Ongoing Weight Loss Phase

As you approach your weight loss goal, you can consume more carbohydrates. Start transitioning from the initial phase of the nutrition plan to the Ongoing Weight Loss (OWL) phase when you are within 10 pounds of your target weight.[2] You can transition to the OWL phase earlier if you desire more variety in your diet, but it will slow the rate of weight loss.

Begin the transition by increasing your daily net carb intake to 25 grams. Gradually increase in 5-gram increments by selecting acceptable foods for the OWL phase. Add back nuts and seeds first, and then add berries. Follow these with some select dairy choices, legumes, and high-carbohydrate vegetables and fruits, and then add whole grains last. Add food groups one at a time to test the impact of their inclusion on your weight loss trajectory.

During the OWL phase it is important to determine your personal tolerance for carbohydrates as you reintroduce them during this phase. Your personal tolerance is called the Carbohydrate Level for Losing (CCL).[2] Personal tolerances vary widely among individuals. Some people have a CCL of fewer than 50 grams of carbohydrates per day while others can tolerate more than 50 grams of carbohydrates per day.

At some point in your weight loss journey, you will determine the daily intake of carbohydrates you can tolerate while keeping your weight in a stable range. It is called the Atkins Carbohydrate Equilibrium (ACE).[2] Most people's ACE is 60-100 grams of carbohydrates, although some people can tolerate more or less than this range and maintain a stable weight. While some people can maintain their weight indefinitely on a LCHF nutritional plan,[2] others find it helpful to change to another nutritional plan that is easier to live with for maintaining their weight. This will be discussed more in Chapter Nine.

Frequently Asked Questions

Since I am eating more fats on this nutritional plan, will this affect my cholesterol levels?

Numerous studies have shown that reduction of carbohydrate intake actually improves fat metabolism and reduces cardiac risk factors by (i) increasing the "good" cholesterol (HDL), (ii) reducing triglycerides, and (iii) changing the nature and/or number of "bad" cholesterol particles (LDL), which appears to render them less likely to stick to the lining of arteries.[2,3]

Can I expect to reduce the dosage of or discontinue some medications as my health improves?

People on a reduced-carbohydrate diet see improvement in their high blood pressure or type 2 diabetes, and are able to reduce the dosage of or discontinue some of their medications as the effects of metabolic dysfunction are reversed. *Any changes in medications must occur under the supervision of your PCP.*

What role does exercise play in this wellness plan?

Being active supports overall health and wellbeing. In the initial phase of the nutritional plan "exercise" is limited to simple activities like walking. Each week the time and frequency should be adjusted upwards as you are able. The goal during this initial phase is 30 minutes of activity 4-5 days/week. Exercising too much during this phase can stall weight loss. Once you reach the maintenance phase, you may introduce additional types of exercises (e.g. cardio and resistance training).

How often should I weigh?

The key to weighing is not letting the number on the scale stress you out (and increase your cortisol level!). You can weigh daily, every few days, or weekly to track your progress. **The important thing is to weigh at some regular interval.** Weighing less frequently or averaging your weight over some predetermined interval can smooth out those changes related to fluid shifts, premenstrual fluid retention, or intestinal weight retention. It is well known that fluctuations of several pounds can occur because of these conditions.

Is it important that I take body measurements?

Yes. Measure yourself every week or two during the weight loss phase for several reasons. Some weeks you may not lose much weight, but you will detect some "loss" from your measurements. Also, calculate your body mass index (BMI) using your height and weight, and your waist-to-height ratio. According to established standards, a BMI over 30 means you are obese, and a BMI over 25 means you are overweight. However, there are athletes that because of muscle mass have BMIs over 30. So in some cases it is not an accurate reflection of one's metabolic state. It has also been shown that increased abdominal girth is associated with inflammation leading to coronary artery disease and type 2 diabetes. These realities make determining your waist-to-height ratio very important. An ideal waist-to-height ratio is less than 0.5.

If I am taking an SSRI for depression and it causes weight gain, are there better alternatives for treatment of my depression while in the program?

Talk with your PCP about changing to Bupropion since it will not cause the weight gain that SSRIs can cause. In addition, ketogenic diets have been shown to help reduce depression.

What medications do you use to help patients lose weight?

- **Metformin** can be very helpful. It has a long track record for safety and efficacy in treatment of patients with type 2 diabetes. It is useful for people with insulin resistance or metabolic syndrome and can be helpful for people with a BMI greater than 30. It has minimal side effects if taken with food. However, some children develop negative gastrointestinal effects, in which case topical Metformin works better.

- **Phentermine** can be helpful for some patients if appetite control remains an issue despite adhering to the diet and taking Cell Press. Phentermine, a stimulant medication, is an appetite suppressant, and is very effective in some patients. Some side effects can prove intolerable, but using a low dose enhances patient tolerance. Like Metformin, Phentermine is inexpensive.

What do I do if I can't tolerate the typical protein sources in breakfast foods like eggs or bacon?

As discussed previously, consuming protein early in the day has some metabolic advantages to assist with your weight loss. As an alternative to the recommended breakfast foods you could substitute a protein shake. Depending on your preference, use a vegetable protein source (e.g. hemp, pea, or a mixture of plant proteins) or whey protein, derived from cow's milk, as good sources of protein. Pick a product that is gluten-free, non-GMO, low sugar (e.g. 2g), and contains 20-30 g of protein/scoop. Mix in 10-12 oz. of unsweetened almond milk. Products sweetened with stevia are preferred.

What are some causes for "stalling" or hitting plateaus during weight loss, and what do I do about them?

- **Medications.** As discussed previously, certain medications can cause weight gain. Inform your online wellness physician of any changes in medication dosage or the addition or deletion of any medications. These changes can affect your progress in weight loss.

- **"Carb creep."** This occurs when you begin to try "alternative" foods or beverages not listed on the diet. It is very important to read the nutritional labels to make sure you do not exceed the daily limit of 20 grams of net carbohydrates. Be more disciplined in tracking your carbohydrate intake. Use a written journal or a phone app to track your daily intake.

- **Eating forbidden foods.** A lapse in maintaining the nutritional recommendations can be corrected easily if it is minor. However, a more significant lapse can be more difficult to recover from (this will be discussed in the next chapter). In the event of a lapse, decrease your net carbohydrate intake by 10 grams, and once the weight loss resumes, add carbohydrates in 5 gram increments as before. The goal is to quickly return to the weekly weight loss you were experiencing.

- **Not drinking enough water.** Inadequate water intake can affect success at weight loss. Make sure you are taking in at least 64 ounces of fluid each day.

- **Not being active enough.** If your energy expenditure is inadequate, your metabolic rate will adjust, and weight loss will slow. Increase your activity to the recommended level and frequency to resume weight loss.

- **Exercising too much.** If your energy expenditure exceeds the required intake, your metabolic rate will adjust, and weight loss will slow or stall. Decrease your activity to the recommended level and frequency to resume weight loss.

- **Skipping meals.** It is so important for the "fat burning" process to not skip meals. Skipping meals will cause your metabolic rate to adjust and stall your weight loss. Adjust your schedule to accommodate the need to eat meals at appropriate intervals.

- **Not eating enough.** If your body's metabolic demands are not being met, your metabolic rate will drop, slowing weight loss. Adequate protein intake to match your activity level is needed to maintain weight loss.

- **Not getting enough sleep.** Inadequate sleep affects your metabolism and can inhibit weight loss. In men, studies have shown that inadequate sleep can cause ghrelin levels to increase, which stimulates appetite and can cause weight gain.[4] Adjust your schedule to try to get eight hours of sleep each night. Develop bedtime routines that promote good sleep habits. Avoid caffeine in the evening, and eat early in the evening.

- **Metabolic problem.** The presence of thyroid antibodies can cause weight loss to stall. If there is no known cause for a plateau, testing for the presence of thyroid antibodies can be helpful because it is treatable and can assist with resuming weight loss. Also, subclinical hypothyroidism can occur in some patients and will impede their efforts to lose weight unless treated. Consider having your PCP obtain thyroid labs to evaluate for antibodies and for subclinical hypothyroidism.

Reaching a plateau in your weight loss is not unexpected and can be overcome. If you continue to experience a plateau despite evaluating potential causes, discuss with your wellness physician. Adjustments can be made that will often result in resumption of weight loss.

Chapter Five

Avoiding Detours

Lapses are inevitable during attempts at weight loss. A lapse is a temporary "slip" in your weight loss efforts and can occur for a variety of reasons. It is important to identify lapses quickly and intervene before they escalate into a relapse. To effectively deal with lapses, identify high-risk situations, and create a plan to deal with those situations.

A relapse occurs when you resume unhealthy eating and activity habits, leading to significant weight regain. A relapse usually results from an accumulation of small lapses. By being preemptive and acting quickly, you can avoid experiencing a relapse.

The path to a relapse begins when a high-risk situation presents itself, and you have no plan for dealing with the situation. An initial lapse occurs. This lapse then leads to negative thinking and becomes a set up for a downward spiral to occur. Another lapse happens if your "damage control" strategy is not activated. Then after further lapses a full relapse occurs.

Identifying High-Risk Situations

When a patient experiences a significant lapse, I give them two worksheets to fill out. The first worksheet (below) helps them identify and plan for their particular high-risk situations.

Use the prompts on the worksheet to guide you as you identify in writing particular high-risk situations that you may face. Then write down how you plan to prepare yourself for the situation or to avoid it entirely:

High-Risk Situations Worksheet[1]

Feelings:　　　　　　Identify-

　　　　　　　　　　Plan or Avoid-

People:　　　　　　　Identify-

　　　　　　　　　　Plan or Avoid-

Time of Day:　　　　Identify-

　　　　　　　　　　Plan or Avoid-

Seasons:　　　　　　Identify-

　　　　　　　　　　Plan or Avoid-

Events: Identify-

                 Plan or Avoid-

Places: Identify-

                 Plan or Avoid-

Weekday: Identify-

                 Plan or Avoid-

Month: Identify-

                 Plan or Avoid-

Responding to a Lapse

The second worksheet helps patients respond to the specific lapse they just experienced. The "S-L-I-P" recommendations that follow on the next page are helpful to use when you are confronted with situations that lead to a lapse:

S-L-I-P Worksheet[1]

STOP

The first step is to stop the problem behavior. Don't listen to yourself — speak to yourself. Take control of the situation by saying "STOP" out loud or by picturing a big red stop sign.

LOOK

It is not always easy to see what happened in any given situation. Step back and ask, "What did I do?" Assess the situation realistically. Be objective and specific in your assessment.

INVESTIGATE

Evaluate the circumstances further by asking questions. What kept you from following your plan? Are your goals specific enough? Are they realistic? Are they achievable?

PROCEED

Write down your new goals and initiate your new plan. Build in some incentives to assist you in achieving them. Get back on track!

Preventing a Relapse

After a lapse, it is important that you take all available measures to prevent the lapse from turning into a relapse. I recommend the following relapse-prevention plan, adapted from *The Eating Well Diet* by Jean Harvey-Berino.[2]

- **Relax.** Recognize that lapses will occur, but it is not the end of the world. It's just a "slip".

- **Resist negative thoughts.** Reject thoughts like, "I'm a failure." Counter these thoughts with the truth about who you are and how well you are doing. Speak to yourself instead of listening to yourself.

- **Evaluate what happened objectively and learn from it.** Identify what happened and what to do about it. Learning from the lapse can empower you to prevent it from happening again.

- **Develop a strategy.** Have a plan for dealing more effectively with high risk situations when confronted with similar situations in the future.

- **Implement your "damage control" strategy.** Regain control of the lapse in eating or physical activity without delay to prevent further lapses. Don't delay.

- **Call for help.** Talk to someone in your support system. Share what happened and your strategy for reversing the lapse. Support from others will help you get back on track with your program.

Staying in the Race

There will be bumps in the road, but you can reorient yourself and stay in the race! Remember, lifestyle change is a marathon, not a sprint.

The Lifestyle Coach Facilitation Guide is an additional resource provided by the Centers for Disease Control (CDC) for relapse prevention.[3] Avail yourself of this material. Arm yourself for the battle, and set yourself up for success.

The battle is not just to lose weight but also to maintain your new weight. The next chapter addresses the challenges of keeping your weight loss permanent. There are many forces working against you, and you need to be aware of what they are and how to deal with them. A good strategist studies his or her enemy.

Chapter Six

Staying the Course

There are no short cuts to long term health; to gain health you have to lose habits. **Losing weight is not the hard part for most people — it's maintaining the weight loss.**

Here is a familiar story: You reach your goal weight, and can now wear your desired size of clothing, but then something happens. Things spiral out of control; you go back to old ways and old habits. This can happen over and over for some people. But don't despair. Keep reading. There is hope. Maybe you are thinking, "What's going to be different this time? I've done this before and ended up back where I started." You *don't* have to end up back where you started. Armed with the truth, *you* can control your destiny.

You "burned your boat," *you* reached your weight loss goal, and *your* health has improved. You are a success! Now you are ready to learn how to stay the course and not regain the weight like most people do. To do this you need to know the science behind weight regain and learn from people who got derailed and lost the ground they gained.

Reasons for Regaining Weight

1. Your body is fighting against you

Probably not what you want to hear. The body has multiple metabolic and hormonal pathways that it can use to restore weight back to a previous "set point." The process is called **adaptive thermogenesis.** This is a scientific term for the body's decrease in energy expenditure in response to weight loss. Doesn't seem fair, does it? However, it is the way we are designed. It's similar to reversion to the mean in statistics or the pressure to stabilize an unstable system. Instability triggers mechanisms designed to bring order and stability back to a system—homeostasis. Weight loss destabilizes the metabolic systems in the body, which triggers complex responses between the brain and other organs in the body to stabilize the affected metabolic systems.[1]

Your rate of metabolism slows in response to weight loss. The body also increases ghrelin levels to stimulate hunger and decreases leptin levels to reduce satiety, or that sense of satisfaction after eating. The body likes homeostasis and will fight for it. There are enough enemies from without that can derail your weight loss success, but this enemy is within and operates 24/7. Do not underestimate its power! It will win unless you work with your body to mitigate weight regain.

2. Life happens

This is the reason I most often hear from patients that relapse. They are doing well losing weight, have made some lifestyle adjustments that help maintain their weight loss, and then—life happens. It can be a relational breakup or divorce, a traumatic experience, a serious illness, or a significant loss. Unfortunately, these kinds of things are inevitable. We live in a fallen world where painful things happen to us or to people we love. How we respond to adverse circumstances is going to affect us body, soul, and spirit. We revert to old patterns of responding to stressful or painful situations. Why? Because these responses are easier, more familiar, or a comfort to us. Unfortunately, these old patterns can adversely affect our health and wellbeing.

3. Lack of accountability

As mentioned previously, it is so important to have regular follow up once you reach your goal weight. Having to check in periodically provides some accountability during the transition from the "diet mentality" associated with weight loss to a healthier "lifestyle mentality" associated with weight maintenance. One large weight loss program in Idaho has shown that it can take up to two years to establish a lifestyle that enables sustained wellness.[2] Regular follow up for an extended time is recommended to ensure maintenance of weight loss.

4. Not reaching out for help when relapse occurs

Getting help quickly when you begin to relapse cannot be stressed enough. It may be asking for help from your accountability partner or wellness group. It may mean getting a follow up appointment *before* your scheduled follow up. It may mean seeking assistance from a counselor or your spiritual advisor. When patients that have relapsed are asked why they didn't come back to the program to get help, they will often say they felt like a failure, or felt shame or embarrassment. You must reject these negative feelings. Reach out to someone for help before things spiral out of control—once that happens, it is harder to get back to where you were before the relapse.

Strategies to Prevent Weight Regain

1. Adopt a weight-maintenance nutritional plan

Many diets that promote weight loss are ineffective in the long run because they rely on unsustainable dietary restrictions, meal replacements, and/or supplements. This can present significant challenges when people try to maintain their weight loss. At some point in your wellness journey, you have to eat a healthy, nutrient-rich diet comprised of whole foods rather than food replacements or supplements. For this reason, it is important to embrace a healthy nutritional plan that you can live with, one that is truly sustainable. Chapter Nine will cover this topic.

2. Increase physical activity

The National Weight Control Registry (NWCR) assessed the predictors of successful weight maintenance.[3,4] Long term weight loss success was defined by the NWCR as a 10% weight loss maintained for greater than a year. Ninety percent of the people in the registry who have met the criteria for long term success exercise daily. The most recent data on the NWCR participants show that a majority of them perform more than 60 minutes of moderate-intensity exercise daily.[5] While exercise is not necessary during the weight loss phase, it is essential to prevent weight regain. The American Diabetes Association recommends 150 minutes of moderate-intensity exercise spread over three times per week as well as strength training two times per week.[6] The American Heart Association and the American College of Sports Medicine recommend 30 minutes a day of moderate exercise five days per week or 25 minutes of vigorous exercise three days per week.[7] A good review of the current recommendations may be found in Steelman and Westman's *Obesity: Essentials and Treament.*[5]

3. Eat breakfast

Eating breakfast is important for weight loss, and it remains important for maintaining that weight loss. Controlling your hunger during this phase of your wellness journey is critical. Eating breakfast and not skipping meals aid both metabolism and appetite control. Eating breakfast was another predictor of success based on the NWCR studies. Of the people who have maintained their weight loss, 78% eat breakfast consistently. Eating breakfast helps jump start your body's metabolism so that you burn calories at a high rate earlier in the day.[8] It can also be helpful to frontload your caloric intake (i.e. eat larger meals early in the day) since you will burn more calories during the day than at night when you are sleeping.

4. Self-monitor

Patients who self-monitor experience greater success in maintaining their weight loss than those who do not. NWCR data show this is a predictor for success in maintaining weight loss. Seventy-five percent of the people in the registry weigh themselves weekly. Self-monitoring might include weighing, keeping a food journal, or tracking activity. There are a number of apps and wearable trackers (e.g. Fitbit, Garmin, etc.) that can be very helpful in monitoring your activity. (See the Resources section at the end of the book for a list of apps.)

Transitioning from the Diet Mentality

Once you have begun employing these weight-maintenance strategies, it's time to take one of the most important steps in your wellness journey. In a sense, you have crested the hill in your wellness journey. It feels great to see your hard work paying off and to have confidence that you can maintain your weight loss. **However, you have not arrived at your destination.** Your efforts are a precursor to the next step in your journey. In some ways this is the hardest but most important step you will take. What you do next can propel you toward your destination—a lifestyle of health and wholeness.

This is not the time to rest, content with your weight loss success, but to press on. Your destination is the place where harmony exists in body, soul, and spirit. The time has arrived to jettison the "diet mentality" and embrace a "lifestyle mentality," to shift from a short-term view to a long-term view. For many people this is difficult because they have operated with a "diet mentality" for so long they really don't know how to make the shift. They would like to make this shift, but they need a roadmap to guide them onto the path of sustainable change.

Sustainable change includes maintaining the weight loss you have worked so hard to achieve, but it is more than that. Wellness involves more than changing what you eat and losing weight; you must change your overall lifestyle. Achieving long term wellness may require a significant paradigm shift for you. But if it allows you to maintain your health, enjoy life, and live longer, won't it be worth it?

Outcome-based medicine looks at successful outcomes as indicators of effective methods or treatments. What is the healthiest lifestyle? What lifestyles are associated with the people who live the longest? We can learn from the healthiest people, and from those who live the longest. What kind of foods do they eat? What are some of the secrets to their longevity? The answers to these questions, along with a template for a proven, healthier lifestyle, are presented in Part Two of the book.

Part Two

———

Embracing a Lifestyle of Wellness

Chapter Seven

Living Healthier Longer

Do you want to live a long and healthy life? Of course. The key is to live a long and *healthy* life, not a long and *un*healthy life. To find out how, let's explore the "Blue Zones."

What Is a "Blue Zone"?

Dan Buettner, in his bestseller *The Blue Zones*, describes a cover story he wrote for *National Geographic* that profiled regions of the world with the highest concentrations of long-lived people.[1] During the mapping process these particular regions were designated by blue concentric circles. The designation stuck, and these "Blue Zones" represented "hotspots" of longevity. How old are we talking about? These areas have astounding rates of people living 100+ years! On the island of Icaria, Greece, Buettner and his team found that one out of three people live into their nineties. These people not only live longer, but they suffer from fewer of the diseases that commonly afflict people in the developed world. **Residents of the Blue Zones stay healthier longer.** While each Blue Zone had its own unique characteristics associated with longevity, there were factors common to each culture.

Since most of us don't live in a Blue Zone culture, it's up to us to make adjustments to our lifestyles that imitate those who live in the Blue Zones. Let's look at some of the commonalities between these cultures, and then consider some helpful recommendations promoted by Buettner to create a Blue Zone lifestyle.

Commonalities between Blue Zone Communities

The following commonalities are what Buettner calls the "Power 9." Each is described in greater detail in his book.

1. Move Naturally

Unlike many of us, the people living in the Blue Zone areas inhabit environments that foster frequent movement. They perform daily physical work like gardening or other labor-intensive activities. They depend less on machines and technology to accomplish their daily tasks, and are much less sedentary than most of us. Their daily activities often involve walking or biking rather than riding in a car, and generally they would not attend fitness centers or gyms.

2. 80% Rule

The idea behind the 80% rule is to reduce your intake by 20% to avoid overeating. This concept is captured well in Michael Pollan's three rules promoted in *In Defense of Food*: **"Eat food. Not too much. Mostly plants."** Limiting your intake will help in weight maintenance, because a reduction in caloric intake is one of the NWCR predictors of successful maintenance of weight loss. The Okinawans, for example, reportedly stop eating when they are no longer hungry, rather than when they are full.[1] The secret here is learning to pay attention to your body. The Blue Zone eating pattern not only involves eating smaller portions, but also placing a larger balance of food earlier in the day. Eating breakfast is essential. Breakfast boosts a person's metabolism and assists with weight maintenance. The typical daily intake for Blue Zone cultures is 1900-2000 calories.[1] The lifestyle nutritional plan presented in Chapter Nine is nutrient-rich and less calorically dense than a Western diet.

3. Plant Slant

A plant-based diet is common among the Blue Zone cultures. They generally eat less meat and more vegetables than someone eating a typical Western diet. Specifically, they eat no processed meat, less red meat, and more seafood than we do. To enhance longevity, vegetables, beans, fruits, and nuts should be foundational to your diet. An American Blue Zone is found in Loma Linda, California among a community of Seventh-day Adventists. Most of the adherents to this faith are vegetarian. Based on population studies, called the Adventist Health Studies, they are some of the healthiest people and have the longest life expectancy in our country.[2]

4. Grapes of Life

Many of the people in the Blue Zone cultures consume moderate amounts of alcohol. While excessive alcohol intake brings known physical and social consequences, a daily glass of wine can have positive health benefits.[3] Because of the known health benefits of red wine, limited consumption of red wine can provide some benefits for your health and longevity.

5. Purpose Now

People in the Blue Zone areas were found to live their lives with a developed sense of purpose. Studies indicate that people who have an expressed purpose for living appear to live longer.[4] Why should having a sense of purpose enhance your longevity? It is about knowing who you are and having a clear vision for your life. Identifying your passions can help clarify your vision. Your passions are those things that get you excited and bring a sense of fulfillment, which can energize your purpose. Having a sustainable purpose is important as you approach the later years of life. It has been said that people who retire "to" something enjoy better health and live longer than people who retire "from" something. It is about having purpose, a reason to live.

6. Down Shift

People in the Blue Zone areas incorporate activities in their lives that help reduce stress. These activities might include a nap, prayer, or social activities. Perhaps practicing the familiar adage "take time to smell the roses" can actually enhance longevity. Since chronic inflammation is believed to promote a number of serious life-threatening diseases, slowing down reduces stress, which in turn reduces inflammatory responses in the body. Anything you do to reduce stress in your life will diminish the response of stress hormones, which in turn will benefit you physically, emotionally, and spiritually. These benefits will produce a healthier, more enjoyable, and longer life.

7. Belong

We were created for relationship. We were designed to live in community. All of the Blue Zone cultures participated in religious communities. Studies have confirmed that observing religious practices is associated with enhanced longevity.[5] The reasons include healthier lifestyles, times of self-reflection and prayer or meditation that reduce stress, membership in a social network, having a purpose for living, and opportunities to serve other people and participate in community-building rituals.

8. Loved Ones First

Prioritizing family characterizes all Blue Zone cultures. They value family and togetherness, and this provides a foundation on which they build other relationships. Older people who live in multigenerational homes are generally healthier and have better cognitive and social skills than those who live alone or in institutional facilities. Living together creates opportunity for communication, for connectedness, and for younger generations to serve and care for the older members of the family. Taken together, this interconnectedness leads to a greater quality of life and can enhance longevity.

9. Right Tribe

Blue Zone cultures consist of communities that nurture a healthy lifestyle through shared values and practices. The values of the community are passed on to each generation, providing powerful reinforcement. Involvement with people who share our values reinforces our values and fosters social connectedness, which correlates with enhanced longevity.

Pursuing a Blue Zone Lifestyle

Together these Blue Zone distinctives are the ingredients of a recipe for living healthier and living longer. But how do you put them into practice when you don't live in a Blue Zone? The next chapter will map out your path to a Blue Zone lifestyle.

Chapter Eight

Blue Zone Lifestyle

While it's probably not realistic to relocate to one of the Blue Zone communities, you can cultivate a Blue Zone lifestyle by embracing a lifestyle modeled after these communities. If you incorporate the following wellness prescriptions into your lifestyle, you should not only live longer but live healthier longer.

Preparing for a Long and Healthy Life

Some of the following recommendations are drawn from *The Blue Zones* by Dan Buettner and can help you in pursuing a Blue Zone lifestyle.[1] Each set of recommendations addresses one of the nine commonalities of Blue Zone communities explored in the previous chapter. These recommendations reflect activities common to these communities that promote health and enhance longevity. While some of the health-promoting advantages of the Blue Zones arise primarily from location and community structure, you can nonetheless optimize your environment to cultivate your own Blue Zone lifestyle.

1. Learning to "move naturally"

The key is to live actively by incorporating physical activity into your daily living. It is about creating an environment of built-in activity. What are some ways to stay on the move?

- Perform physical work that you have been employing someone else to do for you (e.g. yard or house work). Make the work a fun, family activity that promotes health and togetherness.

- Identify someone at work or school who will be your wellness partner and come up with some creative ways to increase your activity at work or school. Make it fun!

- Volunteer with organizations that have opportunities for you (and your family) to serve in a way that increases your activity. You not only will derive physical benefits from activity, but will also enhance your emotional and spiritual wellbeing by serving the needs of others.

- Incorporate activities into your daily life that reduce sedentary activity and increase your NEAT as discussed in Chapter One. There are wearable trackers (e.g. Fitbit) that will alert you if you are sedentary too long. Consider using this technology to assist you. Try to do something simple like walking for thirty minutes a day for five days a week. Make it a goal of walking 5,000-10,000 steps each day. Don't get hung up on the numbers—simply increasing your steps daily will be beneficial. Wearable trackers are great to help you keep track of your daily steps.

- If you are able to exercise, incorporate exercises that are a combination of aerobic, resistance training, and balance promoting (e.g. yoga or Pilates). From an efficiency standpoint, certain types of high intensity interval training (HIIT) have been shown to be more beneficial than traditional exercise modalities.[2] Because of enhanced efficiency, utilizing HIIT can enable you to get the same or better results in your exercise regimen in less time.

Moving naturally is not about doing certain activities, but rather about being active. Choose to be active. Be intentional and follow through on your intentions!

2. Implementing the 80% rule

To avoid overeating, plan to reduce your caloric intake by 20%. Think through what adjustments you need to make to implement this lifestyle change. What are some ways you can do this?

- Put reasonable size servings on your plate and avoid second helpings. Establishing this habit will help you avoid overeating.

- Use smaller plates to create the illusion of eating more food.

- Diminish snacking and the extra calories associated with snacking. If you choose to snack, consume small portions of diet-friendly snacks.

- Eating early in the day and while sitting promotes healthier eating habits.

- Eat slowly and eat deliberately as promoted by the Slow Food movement.[3]

- If you still feel hungry at the end of the meal, wait 20 minutes, and the hunger will usually subside. This really works!

Be intentional in your eating; take control rather than being controlled. The old Ben Franklin adage *"If you fail to plan, plan to fail"* is true. Maintaining your weight loss and staying healthy requires thoughtful, long-term planning as well as commitment to the plan. Have a plan, and stick to it!

3. Giving your diet a "plant slant"

Plant-based diets are universal among Blue Zone cultures. The long-term benefits of a plant-based diet are well known. Numerous studies have documented that, in general, vegetarians have longer life expectancies that non-vegetarians.[4] What are some ways to shift to a more plant-based nutritional plan?

- Grow your own food by planting a garden. You know what you are eating, and you get exercise and pleasure from your efforts. Gardening is a great way to nourish your body, soul, and spirit!

- Eat less meat (volume and frequency) and increase your vegetable intake by including several vegetable servings each day.

- Include nuts and beans in your nutritional plan; they provide protective health benefits and enhance longevity.

This lifestyle change is foundational to living healthier and living longer. To assist you, a plant-based nutritional plan is outlined in the next chapter. Eat more veggies!

4. Drinking alcohol in moderation

If you do not have health issues, religious convictions, or alcohol abuse tendencies that preclude alcohol consumption, then consider including alcohol in your wellness plan. Moderation is the key word, though. Consume **limited amounts** of alcohol, since people who consume alcohol in moderation generally live longer than both abstainers and heavy drinkers. Limited consumption of red wine in particular appears to promote longevity. Most people in Blue Zone communities consume moderate amounts of alcohol, often at meals or during interaction with friends. What might it look like to add alcohol to your wellness plan?

- Consume limited quantities of alcohol at social settings with friends, since these are both health-promoting activities.

- Buy boxed red wines, which are more economical and generally better quality than buying large bottles.

- Institutite a "Wine at 5" break and have a glass of wine paired with some nuts for a healthy interlude. It provides an enjoyable transition time between the day and the evening — time to relax and take a breather.

Alcohol consumption, while not necessarily beneficial for some people, can be included in your wellness lifestyle. Take time for wine — it's good for your heart!

5. Living a life of purpose

People who have an expressed purpose for living appear to live longer. What can you do to create a sense of purpose for your life?

- Ask yourself; "What am I living for?" or "Why am I here?" The answers can be very helpful in clarifying your purpose. Having a faith-based purpose can be very helpful because then your purpose is defined by God and not by you. If you have a clear sense of your purpose here on earth, then continue to pursue your destiny passionately. If you don't have a clear sense of purpose, then try adopting a faith-based purpose.

- Take time to evaluate your passions. What are your passions? Do your passions line up with your perceived purpose? Knowing the answers to these questions can help you get on track and stay on track with fulfilling your purpose. Identifying your passions can help fuel pursuit of your destiny.

- Develop a personal mission statement. Start with what you are passionate about, and go from there. Knowing your purpose and your passions can help you pursue your calling in this life.

Sometimes we can veer off the path of life, and must make course corrections to get back on track with our purpose in order to fulfill our calling. Having purpose is like having a compass to guide you and keep you on the right path on your journey. Discover your purpose; let it guide you!

6. Slowing down the pace of life

Management of your time is essential to finding ways to slow down. It is about priorities. It requires evaluating roles and responsibilities and prioritizing them from most important to least important. Guard against the "tyranny of the urgent." To do this requires intentionality and consistency; otherwise our schedules rule us. What can you do to down shift?

- Schedule some down time to rejuvenate your physical, emotional, and spiritual wellbeing. In the Bible it says, "The Sabbath was made for man, not man for the Sabbath" (Mark 2:27). The Sabbath was instituted to provide a day every week to rest from labors, a time to reflect and to focus on God and family. Observing a Sabbath "rest" can help you reclaim some needed time and focus on the things that really matter in this life.

- Create "technology-free zones" by reducing technology or the time spent using it. Overuse of technology can adversely affect sleep patterns, personal wellbeing, safety (e.g. internet predators, cyberbullying), and family communication and dynamics.

- Create some margin[5] in your life. Margin helps buffer against the unexpected things that happen in life so that you are not overwhelmed and stressed out by your circumstances.

Incorporating these suggestions, as well as anything else (e.g. naps, spiritual exercises) you can do to reduce stress in your life, reduces inflammation in your body and promotes your health and wellbeing. Slow down; you won't regret it!

7. Creating a sense of belonging

We were designed to live in community. There are many communities in which we participate: family, religious, ethnic, geographic (neighborhood), social (work or school). What are some things you can do to foster a sense of belonging and build community?

- Find a group that focuses on a particular interest that you share. This is a great way to meet people and develop new relationships.

- Join a social network or support group from which you receive and give encouragement and support. This community could provide an opportunity to develop relationships with like-minded folks who share a common need.

- Consider joining an exercise class or recreational team that not only promotes increased physical activity but can also foster a sense of belonging to a group.

- As mentioned previously, all of the Blue Zone cultures participate in religious communities. If you are not involved in a faith community, consider joining one. Based on numerous studies,[6] it has been shown that participation in a religious community can improve both the quality and length of your life.

Being part of and contributing to a community is an essential component of enjoying a healthy lifestyle. Find a group to which you can belong, and join it!

8. Valuing family

Making your family a priority is very important. What are some things you can do to value and prioritize your family?

- Eat meals together. This can be very challenging depending on your season of life. Family meals foster togetherness since members of the family have time to connect and to communicate with one another. Families that gather for meals often experience a protective effect in decreased substance abuse and delinquency, heightened social wellbeing, and higher academic performance.[7] In addition, sharing together as a family in healthy eating patterns leads to a reduction in childhood obesity.

- Consider group recreational or sports activities that your family can participate in together. This not only provides health-promoting activities for everyone but strengthens family relationships.

- Set aside time for family vacations in order to foster better family relationships. These times away as a family can be especially valuable during the time when adolescents are in the home. Family times can help anchor adolescents during this challenging time of transition in their lives.

- Mutigenerational activities and celebrations are also important in strengthening families and building family legacy. Plan family activities (indoor as well as outdoor) that create a sense of togetherness as well as an opportunity to develop family traditions. Holidays and special observances (e.g. birthdays, anniversaries, graduations, etc.) are great times to create and to reinforce family traditions. These family rituals and traditions can become part of the family legacy that can be passed on to subsequent generations.

Promoting and nurturing healthy family relationships creates an environment for wellness and living healthier longer. Be intentional about your family time.

9. Building your tribe

Interacting with those who share your values reinforces those values and fosters social connectedness. Enhanced longevity strongly correlates with social connectedness. So how do you nurture your tribe?

- Be intentional in your associations with people who share your vision for health and wellbeing in order to encourage one another in this journey to spiritual, emotional, and physical wellness.

- Identify people at school or work that you can partner with who are likeminded regarding health and wellness. Find creative ways to support each other in achieving daily nutritional and activity goals.

- Be purposeful in planning times and activities to spend time with like-minded friends: meal times, fellowship times, and outdoor physical activities that foster health and wellbeing.

- Be mindful of making your tribe appealing to your adolescents. Nurturing a tribe can be very important when your children are in their adolescent phase, when peer approval is so important to them.

As you consider the concept of creating and valuing your tribe, be sure you consider and welcome others into your tribe. Like your family, value your tribe!

A Prescription for Wellness

This prescription for wellness is a proven plan that you can live with—and live longer! If you want to live a healthier life and add "healthy life-years" to your life,[8] then reject an unhealthy Western diet[9] and lifestyle and eat and live like the people living in the Blue Zone areas. The next chapter provides a nutritional plan that incorporates many of the ingredients found in the diets of the people living in these longevity hot spots.

Chapter Nine

A Nutritional Plan You Can Live With

The following nutritional plan incorporates recommendations from *The Blue Zone Solution*,[1] *Grain Brain*,[2] and the MIND diet.[3] It is a Mediterranean-type diet, which has been shown to reduce obesity, heart disease, diabetes, cancer, as well as dementia.[3,4,5] Compared to the low-inflammatory, LCHF nutritional plan used to promote weight loss, this plan is more plant-based and includes more complex carbohydrates. Caloric intake is also reduced to help maintain weight loss.

A Sustainable Nutritional Plan

Foods to Eat Often:

Vegetables: Eat lots of vegetables daily, especially leafy green ones—some of the best of the longevity foods. Cruciferous vegetables (e.g. broccoli, kale, cauliflower, etc.) contain sulforaphane, which has been shown to have anti-inflammatory, anticancer, and neuroprotective benefits.[6] Examples: broccoli, kale, spinach, tomatoes, cauliflower, onions, carrots, cucumbers, Brussels sprouts, etc.

Fruit: Eat fruit frequently, but pay attention to the fruit's glycemic load and eat more fruit with lower (<10) glycemic loads like berries. This will keep you from consuming an excess of carbohydrates. In addition, berries contain antioxidants, which are known to be beneficial for preventing heart disease, cancer, and dementia. Blueberries in particular contain anthocyanins, which promote brain health by stimulating production of "brain-derived neurotrophic factor" (BDNF). It is recommended that you consume the most colorful fruits/vegetables since the "pigment is the antioxidant."[6] Examples: strawberries, blueberries, pears, apples, oranges, peaches, melons, kiwi.

Legumes: Legumes are a great source of plant-based protein and should be consumed frequently. They are high in fiber and phytates, and promote longevity by reducing risk for stroke and certain cancers. They have been shown to have beneficial effects on weight control, insulin sensitivity, and cholesterol levels.[6] Examples: beans, peas, chickpeas, lentils.

Whole grains: Whole grains should be consumed on a regular basis because the presence of fiber in the diet helps reduce cancer, diabetes, and cardiovascular disease.[6] However, some studies report negative health consequences of gluten in our diets.[2] For this reason you may want to consider only consuming gluten-free grains. Examples: whole oats, brown rice, quinoa, buckwheat.

Nuts: Nuts offer health benefits and promote longevity. Rich in antioxidants, nuts also provide cardioprotective and neuroprotective effects.[6] They make a great addition to salads and serve well as a daily snack. Consume frequently, but check their carbohydrate content because some nuts contain more carbohydrates than others. Examples: almonds, walnuts, Brazil nuts, hazelnuts, Macadamia nuts, cashews.

Olive Oil: Olive oil should be your primary oil for cooking and for dressings and condiments. It is beneficial for preventing heart disease.

Garlic, other spices and herbs: Use these as condiments to obtain health benefits. Spices are well known for their high antioxidant content—the more colorful, the better![6] The pigment curcumin, found in the spice turmeric, has been shown to reduce the risk of a number of disorders, including various cancers and several inflammatory diseases like rheumatoid arthritis and inflammatory bowel disease.[6] Examples: turmeric, ginger, cilantro, dill, peppermint.

Seeds: Seeds contain concentrated amounts of vitamins, antioxidants, and minerals, including omega-3 fatty acids. There are studies showing anticancer effects with flaxseeds.[6] They also are a great source of healthy fats—a perfect alternative for people with nut allergies. Add to salads and consume as a daily snack. Examples: sunflower seeds, chia seeds, pumpkin seeds, flaxseeds.

Seafood: Fish (non-farmed) and other types of seafood should be consumed 2-3 times a week. Fish have high levels of omega-3 and have protective effects on the heart and the brain.

Eggs: Eggs are a great source of protein and other essential vitamins and nutrients like choline which supports brain health. Consume only eggs obtained from free range chickens to maximize health benefits.

Foods to Eat in Limited Quantities:

Tubers: Minimize consumption of potatoes, yams, turnips, sweet potatoes, etc., because of their glycemic indices.

Poultry: Limit consumption to 2-3 times a week. Organic poultry is preferred. Rely more on plant-based sources to get an adequate amount of dietary protein.

Cheese and yogurt: Minimize dairy products based on cow's milk to reduce intake of lactose (sugar). Consider instead consuming cheese or yogurt derived from grass-fed goats or sheep (e.g. Greek feta). Goat's milk contains lactase, an enzyme, which breaks down lactose.

Foods to Eat on Rare Occasions:

Red meat: Eat red meat (from grass-fed animals) occasionally. Consider limiting red meat to celebratory meals and other special occasions.

Foods to Avoid:

Added sugar: Sugar-sweetened beverages and juices, processed foods with refined sugars, etc.

Processed meats: Sausages, bacon, hot dogs, etc.

Refined grains: White bread, refined wheat pasta, etc.

Refined oils: Soybean, canola, cottonseed, etc.

Trans fats: Margarine and certain processed foods (read labels!).

Miscellaneous processed foods: Low-fat and "diet" foods and beverages.

Beverages:

Water: Water is an essential component in a healthy diet. Consuming 6-8 glasses daily is ideal.

Wine: Red wine consumed in moderation is shown to have health benefits.

Coffee and tea: Coffee has known antioxidant effects. Green tea has also been shown to assist with weight loss. Limit caffeine consumption to the early part of the day. Many herbal teas offer health benefits and can be consumed in the evening (peppermint, rooibos, chamomile, etc.)

Milk: Because of concern that consumption of cow's milk may be associated with an increased risk of cancer, particularly prostate cancer,[6] consider substituting unsweetened almond or coconut milk. These two drinks are known to provide anti-inflammatory health benefits.

Healthy Mediterranean-Type Snacks:

- Raw vegetables like carrots or celery

- Some nuts or seeds

- Greek yogurt

- Small portion of a leftover

- Piece of cheese

For recipes that allow you to make delicious meals that fit this nutritional plan, consult *The Blue Zone Solution* and *Grain Brain*. Both books contain a wealth of recipes for tasty meals.

Frequently Asked Questions

How do I transition from a LCHF, animal-protein-based diet to a plant-based, Mediterranean-type diet?

At this point in the wellness program you have reached your ACE[7] and are maintaining your weight loss. You have accomplished this by slowly adding back carbohydrates into your diet. Don't panic: these carbohydrates (and others) are permissible in the Mediterranean-type nutritional plan. The challenge will be to continue to monitor your carbohydrate intake as you transition into this new nutritional plan. **Try to limit your carbohydrate intake to around 60 grams each day to maintain your weight.** Some weight gain is acceptable, but you must monitor your intake carefully during the transition period. A slight weight gain can be tolerated in favor of the additional health benefits long term. The biggest challenge for most people is transitioning from animal-based protein sources to plant-based protein sources.

The first step is to reduce red meat (beef and pork) intake by substituting fish, poultry, and plant-based protein sources. Start by adjusting your daily consumption of animal protein and then adjust your weekly consumption over time. Ideally, try to reduce meat intake to 2-3 times a week and reduce the volume as well. Over time, you can reduce consumption to the recommended frequency and quantities. Fish is an ideal substitution. All of the Blue Zone communities consume non–farmed fish. In each case, substitute plant-based proteins (e.g. bean, tempeh, or tofu) as the transition takes place.

How do I reduce my caloric intake to a healthy range?

Dan Buettner offers several helpful suggestions to assist in reducing caloric intake.[1] As during your weight-loss phase, eat a large breakfast and eat only three meals a day. Consume more calories earlier in the day and eat smaller portions at lunch and dinner. For some, this requires planning ahead in order to make adjustments in your meals. Minimize snacking to reduce consumption of excess calories. During family or group meals serve food from the counter and avoid family-style eating to reduce caloric intake. A modest reduction in food consumption is an important part of the lifestyle change that can help ensure sustainable weight maintenance and a healthier, longer life!

How does sleep affect my health and longevity?

Numerous studies have shown that inadequate sleep and sleep dysfunction can affect many systems in our bodies.[8] Sleep habits can affect both food consumption and metabolism because of effects on hunger and satiety hormones. One study showed that sleep deprivation caused a significant decrease in the levels of the hormone leptin.[9] This reduction in leptin stimulates appetite, which leads to weight gain. Inadequate sleep impairs our ability to deal with stress and our resistance to infections. Sleep dysfunction has also been associated with an increased risk of dementia.[10] While you should try to get eight hours of sleep a night, have a goal of sleeping a minimum of seven hours a night. To reach your nightly goal and optimize your sleep, create a sleep-favorable evening time. You can do this by establishing a regular bedtime routine, by eliminating caffeine, nicotine, and alcohol in the evening, by avoiding late suppers, and by limiting technology in the bedroom. Exposure to the light generated from electronic devices can have effects on our brains that can interfere with restful sleep.[11]

Are there other interventions that can improve my health and enhance longevity?

Fasting for various periods of time or during certain observances is often associated with the practices of various religious groups. Besides the spiritual benefits obtained from fasting, **intermittent fasting** has been shown to yield significant health benefits, including weight loss, improved insulin sensitivity, reduced blood pressure and cholesterol, and improved digestive function.[12] Fasting may even slow the aging process and reduce the development of dementia.[13] Fasting to help prevent dementia is discussed further in Chapter Ten.

There are different types of fasts (e.g. water only, liquid only, or partial fasts). Fasting can be done for various periods of time (e.g. 12, 24, 48, or 72 hours). Because of the health benefits it yields, consider practicing intermittent fasting, which is an overnight fast for 14-16 hours. After you eat supper, do not eat any food until late morning the following day. I have found that intermittent fasting can be particularly helpful for some patients who are experiencing a prolonged plateau in their weight loss. However, if you have any serious health issues that might preclude fasting, make sure to consult your PCP before attempting a fast.

Adding "Healthy Life-Years"

If you incorporate the recommendations of previous chapters into a lifestyle of wellness, they should position you to enjoy longevity of health. I think most of us would agree that we don't want to just live longer, but we also want to have a meaningful quality of life. By making these adjustments in your lifestyle, you can not only increase your life expectancy but also add "healthy life-years"[14] as you approach your destination. The next chapter addresses an important aspect of quality of life: aging and brain health.

Chapter Ten

Maintaining a Healthy Brain

This chapter addresses how to protect brain health and cognitive function during the final phase of your wellness journey. You have run your race well so far: let's finish well.

Neurologist Dr. Richard Restak writes, "Until the day we die our brain remains capable of change, according to the challenges that we set for it."[1] The direction those changes in our brains take us can be positive or negative, depending on the challenges. Over our lifetimes our brains are met with many challenges from within (genetic) and without (diet and environment). Our brains face constant nutritional, infectious, and toxic challenges. The neuroprotective design of the blood-brain barrier and the plasticity of the brain and central nervous system are truly remarkable. That so many of us function so well for so long is amazing. However, because of genetic predisposition and/or a breakdown in the neuroprotective defenses in our bodies, we can suffer a variety of neurological or neurodegenerative diseases. Some of these diseases manifest early in life (e.g. autism) while others manifest as we get older (e.g. multiple sclerosis, Parkinson's disease, and Alzheimer's disease).

Many of these disorders are incurable, and treatments generally fail to significantly alter the course of the disease (e.g. Parkinson's, Alzheimer's, and amyotrophic lateral sclerosis — ALS). For patients diagnosed with these disorders, hope for reversal of symptoms remains elusive. Efforts over many years by pharmaceutical companies to develop effective medications to treat these diseases have disappointed. However, new research is showing reversal of symptoms in some patients afflicted with these diseases.[2,3] Innovative research shows promising results in treating some neurodegenerative diseases associated with aging, particularly Alzheimer's. This is encouraging because Alzheimer's is the third leading cause of death in the United States. The 2017 annual report of the Alzheimer's Association says that every 66 seconds someone in the U.S. develops Alzheimer's disease, and by 2050 it is projected that the occurrence rate will be every 33 seconds.[4] Additionally, they predict that by 2050 more than half of all Americans over the age of 65 will have Alzheimer's disease. For every patient diagnosed, there is one (or more) care giver affected. These are sobering statistics, especially when you consider the physical, emotional, and financial impact.

To address some of the issues related to these neurodegenerative diseases, let's discuss the role of inflammation, how to screen for potential problems, as well as what nutritional and nutraceutical interventions can be used for prevention or treatment. The information presented augments the nutritional and lifestyle recommendations offered in prior chapters to promote "healthy life-years" during the aging process.

Inflammation and the Brain

Dr. David Perlmutter in his book *Grain Brain* discusses how various components in our diets can compromise brain health.[2] Specifically, he cites studies indicating that gluten and a high-carbohydrate diet promote chronic inflammation in our bodies, leading to a number of inflammatory disorders like type 2 diabetes, cancer, cardiovascular disease, and neurodegenerative diseases like Parkinson's and Alzheimer's. Inflammation occurs in response to some stress on a system. In this case, as a result of inflammation, oxidative stress occurs, causing an increase in production of free radicals in tissues. In response to the presence of free radicals, cytokines (cytotoxic chemicals) are released in the body, and they are toxic to cells in various organs, including our brains.

It has been known for some time that if you have diabetes you are at increased risk to develop Alzheimer's disease.[5] What's the relationship? Chronic intake of sugar in our diets leads to elevated levels of blood glucose (sugar). In response to a rise in blood sugar the body has to produce more insulin. Unchecked, this condition leads to insulin resistance and eventually to development of type 2 diabetes. The inability of the body to properly handle the elevated levels of blood glucose results in inflammation and oxidative stress in the brain. This inflammation alters neurotransmitter levels and causes glycation, a process in which sugar molecules attach to other molecules (e.g. proteins) in the brain, altering their structure and disrupting their function. This process is believed to result in cognitive decline seen in people with diabetes.[6]

A growing body of scientific research supports reducing inflammation in our bodies by adjusting our diets in order to prevent life-threatening diseases like diabetes and Alzheimer's. By making lifestyle adjustments that assist in preventing a number of these inflammatory disorders, you can add "healthy life-years" and protect your brain.

Evaluating Brain Health

Assess your risk of developing a neurodegenerative disease by screening for metabolic dysfunction that could impair brain health. You may have had some of these labs performed during the initial part of the wellness program to establish a baseline metric before you started on the LCHF nutritional plan. If not, or if you did previously but have not had them performed recently, repeat the labs. Consider obtaining the following labs. (The optimal levels are based on recommendations that will help maintain a healthy brain.)[2,3]

- **Comprehensive metabolic panel (CMP):** This test is a good screen for general metabolic function in several systems. In particular, it will screen your blood glucose level. Normal range: 70-100 mg/dL.

- **Hemoglobin A1C:** This test represents your average blood sugar level over the last several months. It is a better test than a spot-check of your blood sugar like the CMP. Depending on the level, people may be diagnosed as pre-diabetic or as having diabetes. The HbA1C test is used to monitor the control of blood sugars in people with diabetes. Elevated levels indicate inflammation and can harm the brain. Optimal level: < 5.4%

- **C-reactive protein (CRP):** This test is a useful screen for general inflammation. Optimal CRP level: < 3 mg/L.

- **Fasting insulin:** This test screens for the development of insulin resistance (IR), an indicator of metabolic dysfunction. IR precedes the development of type 2 diabetes. Early detection can lead to reversal of IR, preventing the development of diabetes. Optimal insulin level: < 3 uIU/ml.

- **Vitamin D:** This "vitamin" is actually a fat-soluble hormone that has numerous effects on various organs, including the central nervous system and the brain. Besides having regulatory effects on the brain, it is neuroprotective through anti-inflammatory effects. Optimal level: around 80 ng/mL.

- **Homocysteine:** High levels of homocysteine have been associated with a variety of inflammatory diseases, including dementia. Optimal level: < 8 umol/L.

The following labs are more expensive and used to screen for specific abnormalities that can impact neurological function. Discuss with your PCP whether you should obtain any of these labs:

- **Glutamate (amino acid profile):** This amino acid is an excitatory neurotransmitter which, if levels are too high in the brain, can cause deleterious neurological effects. It has been implicated in both Parkinson's disease and Alzheimer's disease.[7]

- **Cyrex Array 3:** This array is a comprehensive panel of tests that screens for gluten sensitivity, which is believed to negatively impact brain health.[2]

- **Cyrex Array 2:** This array of tests screens for compounds associated with intestinal permeability (i.e. "leaky gut"). Numerous studies in recent years implicate the gut microbiome and gut permeability in a variety of inflammatory diseases, including neurodegenerative diseases.[2]

- **Cyrex Array 20:** This array screens for blood-brain barrier permeability (i.e. "leaky brain"). Inflammatory processes can cause breakdown in the blood-brain barrier, leading to neurotoxicity resulting in neurological dysfunction and degeneration.

- **ApoE4:** Dr. Dale Bredesen recommends screening for this gene associated with Alzheimer's disease.[3] Consider having this test done if you have a positive family history for Alzheimer's, or if you or a loved one has cognitive impairment or dementia. Knowing whether you have the gene helps you determine your risk of developing Alzheimer's. With Dr. Bredesen reporting reversal of cognitive impairment with intervention, early intervention may delay onset of or reverse cognitive impairment.

Neuroprotective Interventions for Brain Health

1. Nutrition

Eating a low-inflammatory diet is essential to nurturing a healthy brain. A low-inflammatory diet such as a LCHF diet or Mediterranean-type diet as presented in this book provides the foundation for promoting brain health. If you do not embrace a brain-friendly diet, you will limit the effectiveness of other neuroprotective interventions. If you have not made the necessary adjustments in your diet to optimize brain health, take these measures now to prevent neurological dysfunction and cognitive impairment as you add "healthy life-years."

2. Fasting

Numerous studies have demonstrated that fasting yields favorable health benefits, including slowing aging and the development of dementia.[8] Fasting has been reported to yield neuroprotective benefits by increasing brain-derived neurotrophic factor (BDNF) as well as stimulating the Nrf2-antioxidant pathway, which produces neuroprotective factors.[2] One study used 12-hour overnight fasting in the treatment of patients with cognitive decline.[3]

3. Exercise

You know the importance of incorporating regular exercise into your lifestyle to maintain your weight and to enjoy other health benefits. Exercise also provides numerous benefits for the brain that can help prevent cognitive impairment.[2] These include improving memory, reducing inflammation by increasing insulin sensitivity and activating the Nrf2 pathway, and increasing BDNF levels, which promotes neurogenesis or the growth of new brain cells. One study showed that sedentary people are at a significantly higher risk of developing Alzheimer's disease than people who are active.[9]

4. Supplements

While optimizing your diet by consuming whole foods will help you obtain many nutrients essential for brain health, several studies report that certain supplements appear to provide neuroprotective benefits.[2,3] With increasing numbers of people being diagnosed with dementia, supplementation with certain nutraceuticals should be considered. The recommended doses are found in the two sources cited.

- **Curcumin:** The active ingredient in turmeric, a spice, has been reported to increase BDNF, which appears to promote neurogenesis as well as yield neuroprotective effects.[2] It has been used to treat patients experiencing cognitive decline due to its anti-inflammatory properties as well as to reduce B-amyloid accumulation associated with Alzheimer's disease.[3] Recommended dose: 350 mg 1-2 times a day.

- **Resveratrol:** A natural ingredient in red wines, resveratrol has been shown not only to promote heart health, but also to enhance blood flow in the brain, increase BDNF levels, and encourage longevity by activating certain genes.[2] It has been used to treat people demonstrating cognitive decline.[3] Recommended dose: 100 mg twice a day.

- **Probiotics:** These living organisms promote healthy gut-brain communication. Probiotics reduce stress and anxiety while having positive effects on neurotransmitter function.[2] They have been used to treat people exhibiting symptoms of cognitive decline.[3] Recommended dose: 1 capsule daily containing 10-20 billion active bacteria per capsule (includes a variety of strains). Additional information is found in Chapter Three.

- **DHA (docosahexaenoic acid):** This omega-3 fatty acid found in fish, algae, flaxseed, and avocado has well-known anti-inflammatory and neuroprotective effects, increasing BDNF levels and activating the Nrf2 antioxidant pathway.[2] It has also been used as part of a treatment plan for patients with dementia.[3] Recommended dose: 750-1000 mg daily.

- **Vitamin D:** Deficiency in this hormone has been associated with cognitive decline,[2] and it has been used in the treatment of patients experiencing cognitive decline.[3] Recommended dose: 5,000 IU daily of Vitamin D3.

- **Alpha-lipoic acid:** This fatty acid provides energy along with antioxidant effects. These effects are neuroprotective and may be useful in treatment of dementia.[2] Recommended dose: 600 mg daily.

- **MCT oil (coconut oil):** Coconut oil serves as a great energy source and appears to be useful in preventing and treating neurodegenerative disease.[2,3] It has known anti-inflammatory benefits as well. Recommended dose: 1 Tbsp. daily.

Continuing Your Journey

If you have read everything up to this point and initiated the program, you should be well into your wellness journey. You have received a roadmap for weight loss, for weight maintenance, for sustainable and healthy lifestyle changes, and for maintaining a healthy brain during the aging process. Hopefully, you are experiencing many of the health benefits accrued from these changes in your lifestyle. Some of you have experienced reversal of weight-related disorders. You are to be commended for your persistence in your efforts! Don't rest on your accomplishments, however, but be ever vigilant to maintain your success. There is no coasting on this journey. It is a lifelong endeavor and well worth it. Fight the fight, and even if you lose a battle here or there, don't look back. Stay in the race! Keep running for the finish line while keeping your eyes on the prize.

Epilogue

A Prescription for Wholeness

Following the recommendations in this book will yield lasting results: a new outlook with a new lifestyle that allows you to live healthier longer. But there's more to human existence than the physical body. I want to challenge you to look beyond your physical and emotional health and pursue wholeness. I believe that, until we experience wholeness in body, soul, and spirit, we will not experience lasting wellness.

The operating principle of my practice is captured well in the words of Johann Wolfgang von Goethe:

If we treat people as they are, we make them worse. If we treat people as they ought to be, we help them become what they are capable of becoming.

I want to help people become what they ought to be — the whole persons God created them to be. Wholeness is derived from a balanced integration of body, soul, and spirit. So how do you experience this wholeness? It begins by knowing who you are, and what your purpose is. Let me tell a story that illustrates this path to wholeness.

***

Three co-workers, Govinda, Olivia, and Dan, form a wellness group to encourage one another and provide accountability to reach their wellness goals. Like most people they have had their successes and their inevitable lapses during their journey together. They all are committed not just to losing weight, but also to forming habits that will enable them to live healthier longer.

This wellness group has enabled them to develop great relationships and to get to know one another better. They have shared their stories, their hopes, and their dreams with one another. During the course of this journey another co-worker, without warning, has a heart attack at home and dies. The suddenness of his death shakes everyone. He was a husband, a father of two, and a valued colleague. They each wonder. *Why did this happen? Why did he die so young?* This death interrupts their journey and confronts the three co-workers with their own mortality. More questions follow: *Why are we here? Do our lives really matter? What happens when we die?"*

After the funeral for their friend, they go out for drinks. Their conversation quickly turns to the weighty questions provoked by death.

Govinda recognizes the sense of identity that religious practices can bring. His family's cultural observance of their religion carried him through childhood. But this identity faded as he reached adulthood and left home. "We are here," he now tells his co-workers, "as the result of a random series of events in the long chain of human evolution. Our identities come from the choices we make. My education, my work, my family— that's where I find the meaning of life. That's all there is— you're born, you make the most out of your life, and at some point you die. End of story."

Olivia, on the other hand, grew up in a non-religious home, but her spiritual interests awakened in high school and heightened during college. Her eclectic spirituality involves prayer and meditation as well as participation in a spiritual community. She affirms Govinda's pursuit of meaning in life but adds in another concept: God. "We are all from God and a part of God," she says. "And God is in each of us. Our purpose in life is to participate in the divine, to make the divine real in our lives and in the lives of others."

"If the divine even exists," asks Govinda, "How do you find it?"

"Where there is love," Olivia answers, "there is God. When you love yourself by doing what brings you happiness, and when you connect with other people, like we're doing now, you find God. God is the impulse of love that energizes the Universe. And when we die, our own energy rejoins the divine."

Dan jumps in and asks, "Do you see God as a person—a person who created us and wants a relationship with us?"

"Not in the sense that you or I am a person," she replies. "God is a collective consciousness that connects us all. It's in *our* choices that *we* make God real and give meaning to our lives."

Dan was raised in a family that was religious and went to church regularly. After abandoning the faith and practices of his family in college, he had a spiritual encounter that led him to become a follower of Jesus Christ. He tells his co-workers, "I have experienced God as a person. I have sensed Him call me to find myself in the bigger story that He is writing in human history—a story that rights the wrongs of this world. I believe that God became a human being in the form of Jesus Christ, who healed the sick, whose teachings have been preserved in the Bible. When I look around the world, I see so much brokenness that I can't fix—in the sadness of death, in the sufferings that come from injustice, broken relationships, and disease. I can't imagine finding my purpose within myself—I need someone greater than myself to give me hope in this world."

Govinda responds, "I get what you mean about how messed up the world is, but how can you even know any of this stuff about God is true?"

"Govinda, it's a matter of faith. The story of the God of the Bible makes sense of my life and of the world around me. The Bible promises life after death to all who place their faith in Jesus. I draw a great deal of hope and a sense of destiny by believing that there's a larger plan to heal this world and by being part of a community of other people who believe this— my church."

"I find a lot of strength in my faith community, too," adds Olivia. "And both of you give me strength and hope—I'm so glad we don't have to walk this journey alone."

***

As you read the story, did you find yourself identifying with any of the characters? You may have asked yourself the same questions: Who am I? Why am I here? What will happen when I die? If you are uncertain about the answers, you are not alone!

Not having an established identity, lacking a clear sense of purpose, or being uncertain about what happens when you die can produce all sorts of emotions: fear, anxiety, disappointment, anger, depression, despair. These emotions can have adverse effects on you physically, emotionally, and spiritually. If these emotions are not addressed, they can affect your health and longevity.

In chapters seven and eight, having a purpose for living is one of the characteristics of people living in Blue Zone communities that accounts for their longevity. Having an established identity and clear purpose can anchor us as we weather the challenges of life, like the sudden death of a friend or loved one. I believe that to experience lasting wellness it is important for you to know who you are and why you are here. If you are uncertain about your identity, your purpose, or the afterlife and are experiencing some of these emotions, what can you do about it?

Be intentional in finding answers to the questions of who you are and why you are here. This will help relieve negative emotions derived from uncertainty so you can live a more meaningful and longer life. To assist you in your quest for answers, consider becoming part of a faith-based community of people who share a similar worldview. Becoming part of something greater than yourself is empowering and enhances your sense of purpose. Being part of a community also helps you not feel alone in this grand universe as you live out your purpose with others. As you seek answers to your questions related to identity, purpose, and the afterlife you will discover there is a reason you are here, and you have a meaningful purpose worth pursuing. A balanced, integrated life can occur as you find the answers to your questions.

I urge you to take your spiritual wellbeing as seriously as you take your physical and emotional wellbeing.

If you asked me which co-worker I identify with, it is Dan. His story is my story. Like Dan, I didn't have satisfying answers concerning my identity, my purpose, or what happens when I die until I became a follower of Jesus Christ. It has been a process of discovery and learning how to live out of my God-given identity as I fulfill my God-given purpose.

Many people relate to God (or to their own conscience) as a difficult-to-please taskmaster. They think, "If I do this, and this, and this, God will be happy with me." This performance-based relationship can be burdensome and create uncertainty and anxiety since you are never sure you have done enough to satisfy God's (or your own) requirements for approval. I have found, however, that God reaches out to us by revealing Himself through His Son, Jesus Christ, and through Jesus we find acceptance, purpose and freedom.

If you are interested in learning more about how to have a relationship with God through Jesus Christ, contact me at **drspruill@roanokewellnesscenter.com.** I would love to hear about your journey to wholeness! *May you be in good health, as it goes well with your soul.*

Appendix

Making a Difference

How did I get into wellness medicine? After receiving an undergraduate degree in psychology, I went to graduate school and obtained a Ph.D. in pharmacology. I enjoyed doing research for several years; however, my childhood dream was to be a doctor, so I went to medical school when I was 34 years old. A late bloomer! Upon completion of my training, I started practice as a general pediatrician.

After an enjoyable 22 years of practice, I began to think about my next season of life. I didn't want to retire so much as to transition to something else that I could be passionate about and do part-time. Around this time one of my sons began a reduced-carbohydrate diet and started to lose weight. My wife and I decided to try the diet, and with this radical change in our diets we began to lose weight. I reduced my BMI to 23 in a relatively short time, and my lipid numbers also improved within months. That was almost five years ago, and we have maintained the weight loss and are very healthy 60+ year olds. While practicing pediatrics I had a growing concern about the childhood obesity problem that continues unabated. Like many other physicians I was frustrated with my inability to have much impact on this problem. I read a report published in 2010 by the White House Task Force that shocked me with a dire prediction: **"one third of all children born in the year 2000 are expected to develop diabetes during their lifetime.[1] The current generation may even be on track to have a shorter lifespan than their parents."[2]** This projection was so disturbing that I decided I wanted to help children and adolescents lose weight and avoid the weight-related diseases that would reduce their life spans.

I began to shadow a physician at a local weight loss program, and to take professional courses on how to treat patients who are overweight or obese. I met Dr. Eric Westman from Duke University and decided to adopt the nutritional approach he uses to successfully treat weight-related disorders. Upon my retirement from general pediatrics practice, I established a part-time family-centered wellness practice to help children and adolescents lose weight and improve their health.

An orthopedic surgeon friend referred some adult patients who needed to lose weight prior to their hip or knee replacement surgery. Over time I began to treat more adult patients who had a variety of weight-related disorders. Like the orthopedic patients, many of these people were experiencing some type of pain because of their weight-induced disorders. It was very satisfying to help them lose weight, reverse some of their disorders, and see them reduce the dosages or discontinue many of their medications. What a twist for a physician to be taking patients off medications instead of putting them on medications. I was hooked!

Why this Book?

I wrote this book because I wanted to give my patients a roadmap to envision them in their wellness journey. Also, I wanted to reach out to people who don't have access to a physician-assisted wellness program. Many people can succeed with this wellness program on their own using the recommendations in the book; however, some will benefit from having virtual consultations. Successful weight loss and reversal of metabolic disorders through online assistance has been reported.[3]

"Losing to Gain"

While practicing pediatrics, I had the opportunity to go on several medical mission trips to impoverished nations. These experiences were life changing, and the suffering I witnessed confronted my comfortable, secure Western world view. This increased awareness of the needs of many people in the world stirred a desire to help alleviate some of the suffering. Over the years my wife and I have supported a number of organizations that provide care for people through feeding programs, providing wells for clean water, training programs, clothing, medical care, housing, etc.

I have been given much in my life, and with that comes much responsibility. I want to give back from what I receive. Some call it "profit with a purpose." I plan to give a certain percentage of the profit generated from this book and the wellness program to organizations that care for people, especially women and children. I like to think of this as "losing to gain." As people "lose" weight, they "gain" health, and enjoy living healthier longer. I "gain" from their "loss" by being able to pass along the "gain" to help others. Everybody benefits!

Your wellness journey is not just about you; it can affect other people beyond your own circle of influence. Your efforts can indirectly impact people in other parts of the world. Let that inspire you in your efforts to achieve a lifestyle of wellness. What you do can make a difference not only in your life but in someone else's life. Join me in making a difference!

Acknowledgements

I want to thank my dear wife Suzanne for being a loving, supportive companion over the 43 years of our journey together. I'm grateful for her emotional and spiritual support. This book is the particular fruit of the last five years in our wellness journey together.

I appreciate the support of my four wonderful children and their spouses in this endeavor. In particular, I thank my son Asher for his thoughtful editing of the book. His editing was invaluable and changed how I write. I am very grateful to son-in-law Mike for creating and managing my websites.

I thank my patients beside whom I have had the privilege to walk on their journeys. They have taught me much that I have in turn taught others along the way. I especially appreciate Steve's friendship and prayers for my wellness practice and this book.

I thank Dr. Chuck Shaffer, an obesity medicine specialist, for his mentoring and encouragement when I first became interested in wellness medicine.

I appreciate my friend Paul's encouragement to write the book to share the vision I have for people to live healthy longer.

I am inspired by how he incorporates "profit with a purpose" into his business ventures.

I thank Nathaniel for using his creativity to design the cover for the book. His design captures well the heart of the book.

Lastly, I thank my Creator for creating me in His image and allowing His creativity to manifest through me in writing this book. I would not have been able to undertake this adventure without His guidance and support.

Resources

Books

Berger, Amy. *The Alzheimer's Antidote: Using a Low-Carb, High-Fat Diet to Fight Alzheimer's Disease, Memory Loss, and Cognitive Disorder.* White River Junction, VT: Chelsea Green Publishing, 2017.

Bredesen, Dale E. *The End of Alzheimer's: The First Program to Prevent and Reverse Cognitive Decline.* New York: Avery Publishing, 2017.

Buettner, Dan. *The Blue Zones.* Washington, D.C.: National Geographic Society, 2008.

Buettner, Dan. *The Blue Zones Solution.* Washington, D.C.: National Geographic Society, 2015.

Greger, Michael with Gene Stone. *How Not to Die.* New York: Flatiron Books, 2015.

Lustig, Robert. *Fat Chance.* New York: Penguin, 2013.

Perlmutter, David. *Grain Brain.* New York: Little, Brown and Company, 2013.

Pollan, Michael. *In Defense of Food*. New York: Penguin Books, 2008.

Scinta, Wendy. *BOUNCE™, A Weight-Loss Doctor's Plan for a Happier, Healthier, and Slimmer Child*. New York: Medical Weight Loss of New York, PLLC, 2013.

Steelman, G. Michael and Westman, Eric. *Obesity: Evaluation and Treatment Essentials*. New York: Informa Healthcare, 2010.

Taubes, Gary. *Why We Get Fat: And What to Do About It*. New York: Anchor Books, 2010.

Westman, Eric C., Phinney, Stephen D., and Volek, Jeff S. *The New Atkins for a New You*. New York: Simon and Schuster, 2010.

Websites

Atkins Carb Counter – A resource and carbohydrate tracker for people on low-carb diets: locarbconnection.com/AtkinsFreeCarbCounter.pdf

Blue Zones – Dan Buettner's collection of resources and recipes: bluezones.com

Controlled Carbohydrate Nutrition – Jacqueline Eberstein, RN provides resources and recipes for low carb diets: controlcarb.com

David Perlmutter, MD – The author of *Grain Brain* provides comprehensive nutrition and health sciences resources: drperlmutter.com

Forks over Knives – Resources, recipes, meal planners, and a cooking course for plant-based diets: forksoverknives.com

Hold the Toast – Dana Carpender's recipes for low-carb diets: holdthetoast.com

Ketogenic Diet Resource – Recipes, meal-planning tools, and helpful articles for people on a ketogenic diet: ketogenic-diet-resource.com

Linda's Low-Carb Menus and Recipes – Recipes for low-carb diets: genaw.com/lowcarb

Nutrition Facts – Michael Greger, M.D., author of *How Not to Die,* offers a collection of articles and videos on health and nutrition: nutritionfacts.org

Whole30 – The website for Melissa Hartwig's Whole30 weight loss and healthy living program; check out their Whole30 Approved program as well as their Meal Planning program: whole30.com

Apps

Atkins Carb Tracker (handy for checking carbohydrate content)

Fitbit (useful for tracking activity, weight, water intake, steps, sleep; has alerts to help reduce sedentary activity)

MyFitnessPal (useful for food journal)

Runtastic (useful for tracking running)

Treadmill (useful for recording steps/distance for walking)

References

Chapter One: Preparing for Your Journey

1. Brechner, Irv. *The Mind Diet*, The Idea Factory, New Jersey, 2013.

2. Levine, J.A. "Non-exercise activity thermogenesis (NEAT)." *Best Pract Res Clin Endocrinol Metab.* Dec 2002; 16(4): 679-702.

3. Pollan, Michael. *In Defense of Food.* New York: Penguin Books, 2008.

4. Lin, E.H., et al. "Effect of improving depression care on pain and functional outcomes among older adults with arthritis: a randomized controlled trial." *The Journal of the American Medical Association.* Nov 2003; 290: 2428-29.

5. Krantz, D.S. & McCeney, M.K. "Effects of psychological and social factors on organic disease: A critical assessment of research on coronary heart disease." *Annual Review of Psychology.* 2002; 53: 341-369.

6. Ozier A.D., et al. "Overweight and obesity are associated with emotion- and stress-related eating as measured by the eating and appraisal due to emotions and stress questionnaire." *J Am Diet Assoc.* Jan 2008; 108(1):49-56.

7. Byrd, R.C. "Positive therapeutic effects of intercessory prayer in a coronary care unit population." *South Med J.* Jul 1988; 81(7):826-829

8. Astin, J.A., et al. "The Efficacy of 'Distant Healing' A Systematic Review of Randomized Trials." *Annals of Internal Medicine.* 6 Jun 2000; 132(11): 903-910.

9. Felitti, V.J., et al. "Relationship of childhood abuse household dysfunction to many of the leading causes of death in adults. The adverse childhood experiences study." *American Journal of Preventive Medicine*. May 1998; 14(4):245-258.

Chapter Two: Are You Ready?

1. Brownell, K.D. *Dieting readiness*. Weight Control Digest 1, 1–9. *JAMA* 1990; 285: 2486–2497.

2. Institute of Medicine. "Appendix B: The Diet Readiness Test and General Well-Being Schedule." *Weighing the Options: Criteria for Evaluating Weight-Management Programs*. Washington, DC: The National Academic Press, 1995.

Chapter Three: Nutritional Plan for Weight Loss

1. Westman, Eric C., Phinney, Stephen D., and Volek, Jeff S. *The New Atkins for a New You*. New York: Simon and Schuster, 2010.

2. Pollan, *In Defense of Food*.

3. Hotamisligil, G.S., "Inflammation and Metabolic Disorders." *Nature*. 14 Dec 2006; 444: 860-7. DOI:10.1038/nature05485

4. Taubes, Gary. *Why We Get Fat*. New York: Anchor Books, 2010.

5. Atkins, Robert. *Dr. Atkin's Diet Revolution*. New York: Harper, 1972.

6. Atkins, Robert. *Dr. Atkin's New Diet Revolution*. New York: Harper, 1992

7. Ferriss, Timothy. *The 4-Hour Body*. New York: Crown Archetype, 2010.

8. Perlmutter, David. *Grain Brain*. New York: Little, Brown and Company, 2013.

9. Helmholz, H.F. "The Treatment of Epilepsy in Childhood: Five Years' Experience with the Ketogenic Diet." *The Journal of the American Medical Association*. Jun 1927; 88: 2028-2032.

10. Fowler, S.P., et al. "Fueling the Obesity Epidemic? Artificially Sweetened Beverage Use and Long-term Weight Gain." *Obesity.* Aug 2008; 16(8): 1894-1900. DOI: 10.1038/oby.2008.284

11. Chia, C.W., et al. "Chronic Low-Calorie Sweetener Use and Risk of Abdominal Obesity Among Older Adults: A Cohort Study." *PLOS ONE* Nov 2016; 11(11): e0167241. DOI:10.1371/journal.pone.0167241.

12. Pace, M.P., et al., "Sugar and Artificially Sweetened Beverages and the Risks of Incident Stroke and Dementia." *Stroke.* May 2017; 48(5): 1139-1146. DOI: 10.1161/STROKEAHA.116.016027.

13. Kobyliak, N., et al., "Probiotics in prevention and treatment of obesity: a critical review." *Nutrition & Metabolism.* 20 Feb 2016; 13:14-35. DOI: 10.1186/s12986-016-0067-0

Chapter Four: Starting Your Journey

1. Wing, R.R., et al. "Benefits of Modest Weight Loss in Improving Cardiovascular Risk Factors in Overweight and Obese Individuals with Type 2 Diabetes." *Diabetes Care.* Jul 2011; 34(7): 1481-1486.

2. Westman, Phinney, and Volek. *The New Atkins for a New You.*

3. Taubes, Gary. *Why We Get Fat.*

4. Schmid, S.M., et al. "A single night of sleep deprivation increases ghrelin levels and feelings of hunger in normal-weight healthy men." *Journal of Sleep Research.* Sep 2008; 17(3): 331–334. doi:10.1111/j.1365-2869.2008.00662.x

Chapter Five: Avoiding Detours

1. Adapted from: Kaiser Permanente Center for Health Research. "Weight Loss Program Materials." kpchr.org/wlmpublic/public/common/getdoc.aspx?docid=2C7F85CA-F476-46FD-8EEF-2D9FA7257BCE

2. Harvey-Berino, Jean. *The Eating Well Diet.* Woodstock, VT: The Countryman Press, 2007.

3. National Diabetes Prevention Program. "Relapse Prevention." cdc.gov/diabetes/prevention/pdf/postcurriculum.pdf

Chapter Six: Staying the Course

1. Sumithran, P., et al "Long-Term Persistence of Hormonal Adaptations to Weight Loss." *N Engl J Med.* 27 Oct 2011; 365:1597-1604.

2. Rader, Allen. Idaho Weight Loss Clinic, Boise, Idaho.

3. Klem M.L., et al. "A descriptive study of individuals successful at long-term maintenance of substantial weight loss." *American Journal of Clinical Nutrition.* Aug 1997; 66(2): 239-246.

4. Wing, R.R. & Hill, J.O. "Successful weight loss maintenance." *Annual Review of Nutrition.* Jul 2001; 21: 323-341.

5. Steelman and Westman, *Obesity: Evaluation and Treatment Essentials.* New York: Informa Healthcare, 2010.

6. American Diabetes Association. "Standards of medical care in diabetes—2016." *Diabetes Care.* 2016; 39 (suppl. 1): S1-S106.

7. American Heart Association. "American Heart Association Recommendations for Physical Activity Infographic." heart.org/HEARTORG/HealthyLiving/Physic Activity/FitnessBasics/American-Heart-Association-Recommendations-for-Physical-Activity-Infographic_UCM_450754_SubHomePage.jsp

8. Ferriss, *The 4-Hour Body.*

Chapter Seven: Living Healthier Longer

1. Buettner, Dan. *The Blue Zones.* Washington, D.C: National Geographic Society, 2008.

2. Orlich, M.J. et al., "Vegetarian Dietary Patterns and Mortality in Adventist Health Study 2". *JAMA Internal Medicine*. 8 July 2013: 1230-38.

3. Ferreira, M.P. and Weems, M.K.S. "Alcohol consumption by aging adults in the U.S.: Health benefits and detriments." *Journal of the American Dietetic Association*. Oct 2008; 108(10):1668-1676.

4. Hill, P.L. and Turiano, N.A. "Purpose in Life as a Predictor of Mortality Across Adulthood." *Psychological Science*. Jul 2014; 25(7): 1482-1486.

5. Musick, M., et al., "Attendance at Religious Services and Mortality in a National Sample." *Journal of Health and Social Behavior*. Jun 2004: 198-213.

Chapter Eight: Blue Zone Lifestyle

1. Buettner, Dan. *The Blue Zones*.

2. Heydari, M., et al., "The Effect of High-Intensity Intermittent Exercise on Body Composition of Overweight Young Males." *Journal of Obesity*. 2012. Article ID 480467.

3. Pollan, *In Defense of Food*.

4. McEvoy, C.T., et al., "Vegetarian Diets, Low Meat Diets, and Health: A Review." *Public Health Nutrition*. Dec 2012: 2287-94.

5. Swenson, Richard. *Margin*. Colorado Springs, CO: NavPress, 1992.

6. VanderWeele, Tyler J. and Siniff, John. "Religion may be a miracle drug: Column." *USA Today*. 28 Oct 2016. usat.ly/2eCspv5.

7. Story, M. and Neumark-Sztainer, D., "A perspective on family meals: Do they matter?" *Nutrition Today*, 2005; 40 (6): 261-266.

8. Grover, S.A., et al., "Years of life lost and healthy life-years lost from diabetes and cardiovascular disease in overweight and obese: a modelling study." *Lancet Diabetes Endocrinol*. Feb 2015; 3(2): 114-22. doi: 10.1016/S2213-8587(14)70229-3.

9. Pollan, *In Defense of Food*.

Chapter Nine: A Nutritional Plan You Can Live With

1. Buettner, Dan. *The Blue Zones Solution*. Washington, D.C.: National Geographic Society, 2015.

2. Perlmutter, *Grain Brain*.

3. Morris, M.C., et al. "MIND Diet Associated with Reduced Incidence of Alzheimer's Disease." *Alzheimer's Dement*. Sep 2015; 11(9):1007-1014.

4. Estruch, R., et al. "Primary Prevention of Cardiovascular Disease with a Mediterranean Diet." *N Engl J Med*. 4 Apr 2013; 368: 1279-1290.

5. Martínez-Lapiscina, E.H., et al. "Mediterranean diet improves cognition: the PREDIMED-NAVARRA randomised trial." *J Neurol Neurosurg Psychiatry*. Dec 2013; 84(12): 1318-25.

6. Greger, Michael with Gene Stone. *How Not to Die*. New York: Flatiron Books, 2015.

7. Westman, Phinney, and Volek. *The New Atkins for a New You*.

8. National Institute of Neurological Disorders and Stroke, Brain Basics: Understanding Sleep, ninds.nih.gov/disorders/brain_basics/understanding_sleep.htm

9. Taheri, S., et al., "Short Sleep Duration Is Associated with Reduced Leptin, Elevated Ghrelin, and Increased Body Mass Index" *PLOS Medicine*. Dec 2004; 1 (3): e62.

10. Yaffe, K, et al., "Sleep-Disordered Breathing, Hypoxia, and Risk of Mild Cognitive Impairment and Dementia in Older Women." *JAMA*. 10 Aug 2011; 306 (6): 613-19.

11. Hysing, M., et al., "Sleep and use of electronic devices in adolescence: results from a large population-based study." *BMJ Open*. Jan 2015; 5: dx.doi.org/10.1136/bmjopen-2014-006748

12. Johnson, J.B., et al. "The effect on health of alternate day calorie restriction: Eating less and more than needed on alternate days prolongs life." *Medical Hypotheses*. 2006; 67 (2): 209–11.

13. Mattson, M.P. "Fasting: molecular mechanisms and clinical applications." *Cell Metabolism.* 4 Feb 2014; 19 (1932-7420): 181–92.

14. Grover, S.A., et al., "Years of life lost and healthy life-years lost from diabetes and cardiovascular disease in overweight and obese: a modelling study." *Lancet Diabetes Endocrinol.* Feb 2015; 3(2): 114-22. doi: 10.1016/S2213-8587(14)70229-3.

Chapter Ten: Maintaining a Healthy Brain

1. Restak, Richard. *Think Smart: A Neuroscientist's Prescription for Improving Your Brain's Performance.* New York: Riverhead Books, 2009.

2. Perlmutter, *Grain Brain.*

2. Bredesen, D.E. "Reversal of cognitive decline: A novel therapeutic program." *AGING.* Sep 2014; 6(9): 707- 717.

3. Alzheimer's Association. "Alzheimer's Disease Facts and Figures." alz.org/documents_custom/2017-facts-and-figures.pdf

4. Kiyohara, Y., "The Cohort Study of Dementia: The Hisayama Study." *Rinsho Shinkeigaku* Nov 2011; 51 (11): 906-09.

5. Roberts, R.O., et al. "Association of Duration and Severity of Diabetes Mellitus with Mild Cognitive Impairment." *Archives of Neurology.* Aug 2008; 65 (8): 1066-73.

6. Butterfield, D.A. and Pocernich, C.B. "The Glutamatergic System and Alzheimer's Disease." *CNS Drugs.* 2003; 17 (9): 641-652.

7. Mattson, M.P. "Fasting: molecular mechanisms and clinical applications." *Cell Metabolism.* 4 Feb 2014; 19 (1932-7420): 181–92.

8. Buchman, AS, et al., "Total Daily Physical Activity and the Risk of AD and Cognitive Decline in Older Adults." *Neurology.* 24 Apr 2012; 78(17): 1323-29.

Appendix: Making a Difference

1. Centers for Disease Control and Prevention, National Center for Health Statistics, National Diabetes Surveillance System. "Incidence of Diabetes: Crude and Age-Adjusted Incidence of Diagnosed Diabetes per 1000 Population Aged 18-79 Years, United States, 1997–2004." 2007. cdc.gov/diabetes/statistics/incidence/fig2.htm

2. Olshansky, J., et al. "A Potential Decline in Life Expectancy in the United States in the 21st Century." *The New England Journal of Medicine*, 17 May 2005; 352(11): 1138-1144.

3. McKenzie, A.L., et al. "A Novel Intervention Including Individualized Nutritional Recommendations Reduces Hemoglobin A1c Level, Medication Use, and Weight in Type 2 Diabetes" *JMIR Diabetes*. 2017; 2(1): e5.

Made in the USA
Lexington, KY
25 September 2017